MY CANCER JOURNEY

FROM DISCOVERY TO RECOVERY

PETER GREEN

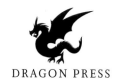

DRAGON PRESS

This is Peter Green's story about his personal journey to the best of his recollection. Some of the names and identifying details have been changed to protect the privacy of individuals. The exercise program provided in this book is not intended as a substitute for the medical advice of physicians. The reader should regularly consult a physician in matters relating to their health and particularly with respect to any symptoms that may require diagnosis or medical attention.

For my son, Benjamin, whose love gave me the courage to fight when I heard the words, "We found something."

For my cousin, John, who battled cancer like a true Spartan warrior. His love of family and friends was always his paramount commitment. He is sorely missed, but his spirit lives on in all of us.

Finally, for my wife Mary. Without her support this book never would have been written. The love I have for her has driven me harder to prove it was worth it.

TABLE OF CONTENTS

PART II: THE EXERCISES

PREFACE: A Sense of Purpose

A few days before Christmas 2005.

I'm collapsed on the couch, recovering from my first cycle of chemotherapy for brain cancer—B-cell lymphoma. After receiving the initial dose through an intravenous tube, I was kept in the hospital for four days of observation until I had peed and puked out enough of the drugs from my body to go home.

It was a brutal few days, but lying here at home I feel a surprising inspiration. I say to myself, "You've got to *do* something!" As weak as I am, my intuition tells me a little exercise will help me get better. So, without really thinking, I roll off the couch and ease down onto the floor.

My first impulse is to begin as gradually as possible. I'll just try a stretch. I lie on my back with my knees bent and my feet flat on floor. I close my eyes. I turn my palms toward the ceiling and take a deep breath. Now I can feel every part of my body. I think about the snow angels I used to make as a kid. I slowly move my arms away from my body along the floor and up and over my head until my hands almost touch. I exhale and take another deep breath. I feel the small of my back pressing against the floor and my stomach muscles stretching and tightening. Despite my exhaustion, this small, slow movement feels great. Then I bring my thumbs and forefingers together in the shape of a heart and gradually raise my hands over my head. I open my eyes and stare at the ceiling through the heart of my hands.

Next, I lower my arms back to the floor above my head and

close my eyes again. I begin to see a variety of colors. It occurs to me I might be able to control the colors I am seeing just by imagining them. "Okay, I tell myself, when I see purple I'll know my body is perfectly aligned."

My mind and body is transported to another world, one that leads to a daily routine of gradually more strenuous exercise. However, I always do them at a slow, rhythmic pace and consider them as much meditation as exercise, as much a benefit to my mental health as my physical. From that first stretch on the floor through my entire cancer treatment, my workout program gave me one overriding feeling: I feel empowered! I have a purpose! This is what I can do to make myself better. This will be my focus. The doctors have their chemicals, and their experimental trials, and their radiation. But only I can decide whether or not to take greater control of my day-to-day routine. And only I have the power to do it.

Within the weeks and months that followed, my newfound commitment made me realize my prior life had lacked this powerful sense of purpose. I hadn't found it at work and I hadn't found it in my first marriage. I larger hopefulness began to emerge. I started to believe I would not only survive cancer, but I could also transform my entire life in a more positive direction. Maybe I could find more meaningful work, become more spiritual, and even change some parts of my personality I had previously failed to honestly confront.

In some ways, I did change for the better and my battle with cancer helped. I fell in love and began a new and successful second marriage. I became even closer with my family and friends. Perhaps I did become a bit more spiritual. But in all honesty, a lot remained unchanged. I went back to the same kind of sales jobs that defined my whole career and I did not really explore new ways of being or thinking. Except for this: for the last twelve years, I've approached exercise in exactly the same way I developed while I was in treatment for cancer.

What I mostly had lost was the intense sense of purpose that had consumed me during that struggle. About two years ago, however, after leaving another unfulfilling job, I decided there might be a way to recovery that focus and dedication. What if I could tell other cancer patients and their families about my experience and how some simple exercises radically improved my morale and my health? Even more, what if I shared the fact that my sense of purpose through exercise made it easier for my friends and family; how it gave them greater confidence seeing my control of the situation and thus made them more comfortable speaking honestly with me? They no longer saw me as a cancer victim or a patient. They just saw Peter, doing what he needed to do.

There are millions of people struggling with cancer today and I hope my example will help many of them gain a greater sense of control and confidence as they work their way through a challenging course of treatment. My exercise routine made an invaluable contribution to my physical and mental recovery and now I want to share it with others. That's why I wrote this book. In doing so, I have recovered a profound sense of purpose.

Writing this book also brought back, with alarming clarity, many of the most difficult and painful memories I had buried. Thinking back on the months of my cancer treatment made me realize how powerfully I had struggled to repress much of what was most real and human about the experience. The more I worked on the book, the more memories returned. Once again, I was transported back to the 7th floor of Sloan Kettering with every sense reawakened. Once again, I could smell the distinct odor of the hospital's disinfectants. I could see the faces of other patients, much older and much younger, walking or being wheeled around the ward, enduring the ordeal of their own treatment. I could hear the tormented voices crying out in the night ("It hurts!" "Where am I?"). I could distinctly remember the strange taste that always formed in the back of my mouth when the chemo began to pour into my veins. And I felt, once again, the sense of helplessness that sometimes overwhelmed me during the endless, nauseated days while I waited for permission to go home.

Recovering those hard memories was as important to this book as identifying the sources of strength and courage that helped me survive. They helped me remember the last thing I wanted during treatment—or that any cancer patient wants—is to be told that fears and anxieties must be ignored. The point is not to ignore them, but to confront them and seek to overcome them, or at least lessen them. Fully acknowledging *all* the complicated emotions that surface during cancer treatment can help people take the necessary steps to make those emotions more manageable and positive after they hear those three terrifying words, "We found something."

PART 1: MY STORY

Discovery

Sunday afternoon, October 15, 2005

I am alone in my home office in Larchmont, New York. Benjamin, my eleven-year-old son, is in the den watching television. My puppy Max, a black-and-white sheltie, is barking at something outside the window. My computer is open to Match.com; at 45, I'm looking for an online date. My ex-wife and I separated more than five years ago and share joint custody of our son. None of these women appeal to me so I decide to click on another page of photographs and profiles. My hand is on the mouse, but nothing happens. I can't seem to move the cursor. I stare down at my hand in disbelief and try again. My right hand won't move!

I reach over with my left hand and pinch the frozen lump. Nothing. I suddenly realize the numbness stretches all the way up my arm to my shoulder. Anxiety instantly pulses throughout my body.

Am I having a heart attack? A stroke? I manage to stand up and wobble toward my easy chair. "Benjamin!" I shout. Despite my panic, I realize the need to get my son. His help may be crucial, but I'm also aware of how horrible it would be for him to stumble upon my comatose body without warning. Seconds after I call, he rushes in. "Ben," I say, as calmly as possible, "If I fall over, you need to get to the phone and call 911. Give them our address." He looks bewildered and scared, but also excited. He knows I'm giving him a great responsibility. He races out to get our mobile phone and returns. "Is it time to call 911?" His voice is trembling. Max bounds into the room and jumps in my lap. "Is it time to call?" Benjamin says again, shuffling from one leg to the other.

"Not yet," I respond. Max jumps off my lap.

"Now Daddy? Now?"

At this point I'm just trying to calm myself and buy time. Take deep breaths, I tell myself. It seems to help. Gradually the numbness begins to lift. I'm finally able to clinch my fist. Ben is still staring at me. "It's okay, son. I'm fine. Really. I just felt a little funny for a while but it went away. I'm sorry for all the commotion. You can go back to your program." He looks doubtful, but my smile seems to reassure him. "Call if you need me," he mutters over his shoulder on the way out. My heart swells with love.

I do feel much better, but I'm worried and queasy enough to do something I'd put off for months. Even after reminding myself that it's Sunday afternoon, with the Giants playing on the tube, I pick up my phone and call my internist—Dr. Silverman. He listens patiently, unperturbed, so it seems, by the interruption.

"First off, Peter, I very much doubt you had a heart attack. If so, any numbness or pain would have been in your left arm, not your right. And by the way, didn't you recently complete a triathlon?" he asks.

"Good memory. I'm actually training for another one."

"Are you lifting weights?"

"Of course."

"Well, my hunch is that you just pinched a nerve."

With that, the tension eases, but only for the moment. "But Peter," Dr. Silverman quickly adds. "We need to check this out. If it were a weekday, I'd send you to the emergency room. But today you'd probably have to wait for hours with no resolution. You *are* feeling better now, *right?*"

"Right."

"Come see me first thing tomorrow morning." He's not overly concerned so why should I be? "Great," I say. "Tomorrow it is." I hang up, feeling calmer. Still, I call my brother, Doug, who lives in D.C. for a second opinion. He's not a doctor, but he shares my passion for exercise. "Could be a pinched nerve," Doug agrees. "But you should probably see a neurologist."

Don't Ignore the Signs

Doug's recommendation triggered a wave of guilt. For several months, I had repressed a nagging realization that I should see a neurologist. I had a long history of avoiding doctors, not because I believed I was so super healthy, but because I always feared I wasn't. Like my father, I suffered from the kind of hypochondria that imagines every imaginable dreaded disease but is too scared to be tested. As a kid, my best friend once told me, "Peter, you do know that you're going to die young, don't you?" I believed him.

In recent months, my fears had a basis in actual symptoms. Months before my arm went numb looking at Match.com, I was at dinner with Heather, my tempestuous, on-and-off again, girl-friend. I reached for a glass of wine and my hand began to tremble so badly I couldn't pick it up. I had to wait a few minutes to make it work. I told myself it was just nerves—my relationship with Heather was fraught with anxiety. Or maybe I just overdid my work-out that afternoon.

A few weeks later there was another flashing red light. I was at a company retreat for Weather Channel executives—I was Senior Vice President of Sales—where we were asked to participate in a series of team-building exercises. In one of them, we had to use our non-dominant hand to draw a line through the pathways of a diagrammed maze leading to an exit. With the pen in my left hand I looked down at the drawing and could see the correct route but could not move my hand. It simply trembled in place. The pen would not budge. People stood behind me cheering me on: "You can do it, Peter. Go on, man!" Somehow, the paralysis passed and I was able to finish my turn. Once again, I ignored the warning sign.

As if that weren't enough, I also became aware that my speech was faltering. I'd be in the middle of a business call and stumble over a simple word and would, like a chronic stutterer, have to think of a synonym I could pronounce. It wasn't denial that kept me from seeing a neurologist; it was fear. I knew something was wrong but didn't want to face the reality.

So, on Monday morning, I finally screw up my courage and call my internist. "I think I should see a neurologist," I tell him. "I think there might be more to this than a pinched nerve."

He gives me the name of Dr. Walkowitz, whose office is on the Upper East Side. I call immediately and make an appointment for Friday. At his office, I tell him about the most recent numbness but not about the other incidents. Dr. Walkowitz looks at me carefully. "You look healthy. It's probably a pinched nerve and nothing to worry about. But I wouldn't be doing my job if I didn't do an MRI on your brain. However, I won't use dye," he adds, as if that were good news.

"Why not?" I ask.

"Well, dye gives us a closer picture, but I don't think we'll need that with you." Eager for every hint of reassurance, I once again push aside my fears. We schedule the MRI for the following Monday—Halloween—and I go home to Larchmont.

That weekend, my older sister, Kathy, comes down from Boston to visit. We are the two youngest of five children and she's the only girl. We've been extremely close our whole lives, in part because I had always looked to her as a kind of surrogate mother and protector. The fact that she's a clinical psychologist makes me all the more eager for her advice on all kinds of personal matters. Kathy and I walk on the beach near my father's home in Westport, Connecticut, and I tell her all about my symptoms and the visit to Dr. Walkowitz. At this point, my habit of denial kicks in and I'm thinking about blowing off the MRI. Kathy is adamant that I follow through. "Peter, look, you can't ignore this. You have to find out what's going on, if not for you, then for Benjamin." Of course she's right.

Halloween morning I call Heather. We hadn't talked in weeks. Our always rocky relationship had been especially volatile recently. I was pressing her to move in with me and she refused.

I couldn't understand why she wanted to remain living at her parent's house on Long Island. In many ways, I was hopelessly dependent on Heather and wanted her by my side for the MRI. However, I didn't want to admit how much I needed her so, instead of just asking her, I beat around the bush waiting for her to make the first step. "Of course I'll come," she quickly volunteers. I had reeled her in once again.

We had been seeing each other on and off for six years. For all our many fights, we each felt a strong bond that was frequently rekindled. In addition to an intense physical attraction, we had dramatically helped each other move our lives in new directions. Heather had given me the psychological strength to leave my first marriage and had helped me in countless concrete ways to re-establish my life, even setting up my computer and organizing my bills.

I, in turn, had helped Heather move upward in the Manhattan business world. When I met her through work I quickly recognized her as extremely competent, savvy, and street-smart. I helped give her new professional responsibilities and opportunities and was eager to cultivate her growth. She was clearly attracted to the more privileged life I represented. At the same time, she was still powerfully connected to her old life.

Heather grew up in a strict Irish Catholic family in a blue-collar community on Long Island. Her father was a New York cop who found comfort at the local bar. Heather had married her high school sweetheart. They had separated but he continued to live very near her parent's home and, for all I knew, she might still be seeing him. All I knew for sure was that Heather refused to divorce him regardless of my pleas. Although I knew next to nothing about her other life on Long Island, I came to see it as a dreaded obstacle to any chance we might have to thrive as a couple. Unreasonable as it was, I wanted her to sever those bonds completely. I wanted her all to myself.

Heather's response was to say nothing about her life on Long Island or to lie about it when she did. She also became even more suspicious of my life. I soon discovered she was getting into my email and catching me in my own lies, especially my denials that I had ever dated anyone else during our intermittent break-ups. I also discovered she had called some of these women and left messages on their answering machines saying that they should have nothing to do with me because I was a "sociopath." As time passed, it became ever more obvious, even to us, that our relationship was, as they say, dysfunctional. Worse still, we were playing out our bad behavior in ways that could not be entirely hidden from Benjamin who had already experienced my failed marriage with his mother. Nonetheless, neither Heather nor I were yet capable of ending our flawed, but addictive, relationship.

We Found Something

In my office, Monday morning, watching the clock, I am still waffling on the MRI. My fear makes no logical sense. I had taken many physical risks all my life. I jumped off high rocks into rivers. I hitch-hiked across country. I worked on a forty-thousand-acre cattle ranch in Nebraska. And for two and a half years I served with the Peace Corps in rural Mauritania. For some reason none of those adventures, however dangerous, caused me excessive anxiety. I always felt I had some control over the risks I was taking. But what could I possibly do if faced with a life-threatening disease? What control could I have over that?

But I know I can't avoid finding answers any longer. Kathy's words are still ringing in my head ("If not for you, then for Benjamin") and I know Heather will be waiting at the clinic. I decide to walk the fifteen blocks to the radiology center. Instead of my usual fast pace, I tell myself to take it down a notch. I'm not going to fight the crowd. I'll just watch the horizon and the buildings that shadow the East River. If I'm going to get through this,

I've got to be more meditative. The frantic New York street crowd begins to fade from my vision and I become more aware that it's a beautiful fall day, with sunlight reflecting off the river. That helps, but I can't ignore the fact that I'm headed for the dark tunnel of an MRI machine and the possible news that my life is in jeopardy.

Heather is sitting in the lobby. After kissing her perfunctorily, I begin filling out forms. She looks over my shoulder. "You're forty-five," she laughs, noticing that I had written forty-six. "Thanks," I say, "You just gave me another year." The joke falls flat. Neither of us smiles.

They take me into the MRI room while Heather waits outside. I see a long table with a tube at the end of it. "Is Doctor Walkowitz here?" I ask.

"Still in his office," the technician says. I'm pissed off because he had promised to be here. They put a mask over my face to stabilize my head and lay me down on the table. Within seconds, I'm sliding into the dark tunnel. "This will take about twenty minutes," says the voice of the technician who is now in a booth outside the room. He'll collect the images and send them immediately to Dr. Walkowitz's office.

Inside the MRI it's even louder and more claustrophobic than I had imagined. The pounding vibrations sound like depth charges exploding around me. I open my eyes to find the ceiling of the tube less than an inch from my face. I order myself to keep my eyes shut until they pull me out of the tube. To forget the walls and ceiling from closing in on me, I try to envision myself as a young boy running across the meadow on my way home from school. I can see the butterflies flitting around me and a startled rabbit bounding out of the wildflowers.

The machine suddenly stops, interrupting my reverie. The technician's voice cuts through the speakers of my metal cocoon. "We need to inject some dye," the voice tells me. "We want a better look." Dr. Walkowitz's prediction proved wrong. I'm surprised by my calm reaction. There is no surge of adrenalin or anxiety.

They slide me from the machine and inject die into my veins. "Ten minutes this time," the technician says cheerfully. I shut my eyes and go back to my peaceful meadow.

At last it's over. The machine is silent and I'm on my feet. I look to the technician and his assistants for information. They are as stone-faced as the presidents on Mount Rushmore. "Do you have an appointment with your neurologist?" asks the technician.

"I guess I do now," I tell him.

As soon as I reach the lobby, Heather hammers me with questions. "Did they say anything?" "Did they smile?" "Are you okay?" She hands me my cell phone. There is an urgent voicemail message from Dr. Walkowitz's receptionist: "Mr. Green, please get to our office as soon as possible." This same woman had been a soothing presence when I had met her for my initial appointment. Now she sounds alien and robotic. I feel a spike of fear.

Walking the ten blocks to Dr. Walkowitz's office every nerve is heightened. I feel a rush of adrenalin that soldiers must feel as they prepare for battle. My eyes pick up even the smallest movements around me. My hyper-vigilance is magnified by the sight of children passing by—ghosts, zombies, and vampires! "It's Halloween," Heather reminds me, noticing my panicked expression.

My ears start picking up the sounds of the trick-or-treaters. "Did we go to this building?" Batman asks his masked friends. A tiny goblin passes us, weeping. Does he know about me? I wonder. "This has got to be a dream," I tell Heather. "I've got to wake up."

At last we reach the office. It's in a brownstone, and the door is already open. There's the receptionist, greeting me with a smile I would see often in the months ahead, a smile that somehow conveys pity, dread, and hope. She ushers me into the doctor's sanctum, Heather following right behind. He comes around from behind his desk and grabs both my arms. "Peter," he says solemnly, "we found six spots on your brain and we're going to figure out what they are."

Silence. I'm frozen in place, numb. "Look," Dr. Walkowitz

continues, "We really don't know what caused this. It may have something to do with your years in Africa with the Peace Corps. You did tell me you had three bouts of malaria then, right?"

"Yes. So the spots could mean anything, right?" I ask, grasping for some hopeful news.

The doctor adds only this. "It's too late to do anything today, but tomorrow morning I'm going to set up an appointment for you with a tropical disease specialist. Call me first thing in the morning, and I'll give you his name."

Looking back, I recall Dr. Walkowitz as a kind man, with sad, soulful eyes. But at that moment, I had gone psychologically numb, unable to let his words, or Heather's worry, penetrate beyond the skin. They could have set me up in a department store window, slapped a suit on me, and I would have been a convincing mannequin.

"I'm taking you home," Heather says. All the tension I felt with her, all the stops and starts, seemed to dissipate with her words. She has a secret life, might even still be seeing her supposedly estranged husband on Long Island, but I am her priority at this moment, and my gratitude is boundless.

Transitioning

Heather makes some whispered phone calls, evidently explaining why she wouldn't be home that night. As we drive up the East River Drive toward Larchmont, my automatic pilot somehow kicks in. I have to let people know my situation. I start with my sister Kathy in Boston. She responds to the news with a long silent pause. She is no doubt quickly calibrating the dire possibilities presented by those six spots.

I'm amazed by how rapidly horrendous news condenses your world. It is powerful enough to block out the sun. But talking with Kathy also makes me realize how much I will depend on a small circle of loved ones; how much I need my own support team beyond the team of doctors and specialists.

Kathy and I agree that it's best not to tell our father just yet. Given his capacity for anxiety he should be brought into the loop carefully. Kathy offers to call the rest of my siblings with my news and asks me to hold on for a second. I can hear her calling out to her fiancée, Chris, asking him to take her boys out for Halloween without her. Normal life is suspended indefinitely, and not just for me. The future is now completely unpredictable.

I call my ex-wife Nancy, whose brother had died of cancer at the age of twenty-two, a painful scar she continues to feel deeply. I must gear myself up, not easy in my perilous emotional state. She's been remarried to John, an environmental consultant, for five years, but because of Benjamin we need to be in close contact and get along as well as possible.

"We don't know what this is," I tell her. "It's going to take some time to figure it out. But I think I better come over tomorrow so you and I can sit down with Benjamin and at least tell him I'm going to be having some tests." We agree this is the best plan.

My oldest brother, Andrew, was staying at my house in Larchmont that weekend after coming for a business trip from his home in Cleveland. He was scheduled to fly home Halloween night, but he had already heard from Kathy by the time Heather and I arrived.

"I'm not going back to Cleveland," he says as soon as I walk through the door. "I want to be with you when you see the specialists." We hug, and for the first time that day, I break down, crying on the shoulder of my big brother, letting every tear that had accumulated as the bad news mounted run down my face. I press my revered brother into my chest, knowing in some unexplored part of my heart that love is a vital medicine.

Searching for Answers

The next morning, Andrew, Heather, and I go to the tropical disease specialist, Dr. Casis. He takes tube after tube of blood, injecting each one into small pre-labeled bottles. He is a taciturn man, just doing his job. I wonder what leads someone to specialize in tropical diseases.

"Do you want me to test you for HIV while I'm at it?" he asks.

"No!" I practically scream. I had been in Africa from 1983 to 1985 at the height of the AIDS epidemic, although I wasn't fully aware of it at the time. During those years in Africa, the disease was spoken of indirectly, if at all. Sometimes people called it the "skinny disease," as if AIDS and starvation were almost indistinguishable. Upon returning home, I discovered the full significance of the global AIDS epidemic. By the late 1980s, AIDS evoked as much fear as the word terrorism does today. Despite every effort to suppress the thought, I always harbored a nagging suspicion I might be infected with the HIV virus. I was in my early twenties during my Africa years and although I was not promiscuous, I was certainly not celibate.

I never got tested. I told myself that the Peace Corps must have checked it out at the end of my tour, but I could never bring myself to verify it. Although I had never experienced any of the symptoms associated with AIDs, I was terrified that a test would come back positive. Now that six spots had been found on my brain the idea that Dr. Casis might also find HIV was too much to bear. To this day, I'm ashamed of my decades-long avoidance of that simple test.

The blood tests came back that day. The good news: I had no tropical disease. The bad news: the doctor still couldn't explain the reason for the spots. I go to other blood-taking specialists, all of them baffled.

Nancy and I prepare to take a seat on the couch to talk with Ben.

Telling Loved Ones

BENJAMIN, 1994

Ben's anxieties may have stemmed from his birth in 1994. He was turned around and facing up as he began to exit the birth canal, causing stress to mother and baby alike. An emergency C-section was performed. I remember standing over Nancy saying, "Just breathe. All is going well," as the doctors literally pulled Benjamin out of her belly. His wailing comforted me. He was alive! But his cries signaled the start of his protest against his new world, setting a pattern for how he viewed his surroundings, especially if anyone tried to tell him what to do.

Until we brought Ben home, the baby in our lives was our dog, Dallas. No longer. As I carried our infant son into the house for the first time, Dallas bounded out to greet me, like a thousand times before. My "Good girl, Dallas," suddenly changed to "Dallas, down!" accompanied by a knee to her stomach. I knew I would protect my son first, forever after.

BENJAMIN, 1999

When Nancy and I divorced, the mediator told us, "The most important thing you must recognize is that you will both be spending less time with your son." Painful, but accurate, words. Ben rotated between his mom's home and my one-bedroom apartment a mile away. Ben recalls those days with me being some of the happiest of his life. Just the two of us, father and son. Ben slept in my room on a big pull out couch. We had a routine. First to Starbucks for my coffee and his milk and cereal. Then to the park to toss the football or shoot some hoops. Dallas always went with us, happy to be the treasured family dog and no longer the only child.

Ben was diagnosed with attention deficit disorder (ADD). That, along with his chronic anxiety helps explain why Nancy and I tended to pamper him too much, without realizing we were enabling bad habits and behavior he needed to outgrow.

BENJAMIN, 2005

On the couch at his mother's side, Ben immediately sensed bad news. "What's wrong?"

"Well," I answered, "I had some medical tests done." I had hardly begun the explanation before Ben interrupted: "Dad promise me that you're going to be okay. Promise. Okay? You're going to be fine, right?" Though he had many questions, and they would continue throughout my treatment and beyond, they were always in search of that original need for reassurance. Often, he was even more blunt: "Dad, you're not going to die, right Dad? Promise me you're not going to die! Promise me, Dad." His terror frightened me, but also motivated me to do everything possible to survive. I tried to make our life as normal as possible. We'd still go out to Starbucks and take walks with Dallas, and when I was too sick to play in the park, we played a kind of mock game of football on our knees in my bedroom.

Now that Benjamin was aware of my situation, his mom Nancy became deeply involved in my care, paying very close attention to my treatment and coming with me on a number of appointments. I'm sure her memories of losing her brother to cancer brought back lots of painful emotions. She is a strong and caring woman and it meant a great deal to have her back at my side. Her family was also amazingly supportive. I'd remained close to her parents after the divorce and her father, Allen, often called me during and after treatment to check up on me.

Never Surrender

I finally decide to drive to Westport to visit my father Paul. At 82, Dad is no longer a magazine publisher, but you would hardly describe him as retired. He is forever planning some new business venture. It doesn't seem to bother him when his ideas are not brought to fruition. His fertile imagination keeps him going. In 1996, at age 73, he had been diagnosed with Parkinson's and from that day forward he was fervently determined to prove that rigorous physical and mental exercise could fend off the disease indefinitely. He became a rower and a gym rat. Now 93, Paul seems to have made his point.

He continued rowing until very recently. I vividly recall watching him a few years ago from the shore of his rowing club. He is shuffling down the dock toward his shell, stooped over and clutching the arm of a young man who had to be 70 years younger. When they get to the shell at the end of the dock, the young man practically lifts my father into the boat. It takes several minutes just to get him settled into the seat, his legs stretched out, and his feet into their straps. The young man finally backs away and my father is alone in the boat on the water.

From my vantage point on the shore, I almost can't believe I am watching the same man who had barely made it down the dock. A magical transformation takes place before my eyes. As he grasps the oars, he raises his head and his stooped back begins to straighten. Dipping the oars smoothly into the water, he pulls the shell out into the river. His body moves with confidence, his arms and legs working in unison. With remarkable skill and grace, my father propels the boat across the calm surface of the Saugatuck River.

Paul is a veteran of World War II. As a Navy lieutenant, he operated a LST that unloaded men and supplies throughout the Pacific, including Okinawa. His hero was Winston Churchill and he adopted Churchill's famous injunction as his own personal mantra: "Nevah, Nevah, Nevah Surrendah!" My father's courage in defiance of Parkinson's has been every bit as impressive as the courage I'm sure he had to muster during wartime. One of the great inspirations for writing this book was my father's many efforts to help others struggling with Parkinson's. He established a "Never Surrender to Parkinson's" foundation to promote the benefits of exercise in forestalling the debilitating effects of the disease.

I am also in Westport to see my step-mother, Eleanor, whom I love not only because she makes my father happy, but because she is wise and loving. From the time I was fifteen and first met her, Eleanor has been my friend and ally. But she isn't home when I arrive. When I enter the house and see my father, it's obvious that Kathy has fulfilled her promise to prepare the way for me by calling Dad to tell him about the spots on my brain. He starts to cry before I say a word.

Though I share my father's determination ("never surrender!"), my own mantra becomes: "Life doesn't stop." Although cancer can be so overwhelming and seems capable of blocking out the sun, you and your loved ones really do have to move on with your lives.

An early challenge is figuring out how to deal with my work. I decide to be as straightforward as possible. I tell my boss and colleagues I'll be having a lot of medical appointments that will take me away from the office but that I intend to do everything possible to keep up with my job. Since we are preparing for our annual national sales meeting, I feel a particular obligation to do my part. And my reassurances make it easier for them to accommodate my frequent absences from the office.

Looking for Clues in Africa

The next step is to consult a phalanx of brain surgeons. Nancy comes with me on these appointments knowing that I need a second pair of ears to recall what is discussed and to ask the tough questions I might avoid. I lug my MRIs from office to office like wedding pictures. The doctors all say the same thing: "Well, you have these spots, but it's unclear what they are. You're in incredibly good physical shape and you haven't had another 'event,' so I've got to think it's something other than a tumor. Tell me again about your time in Africa."

AFRICA, 1983

Nouakchott, Mauritania, a desolate city in West Africa, encompasses a large swath of the Sahara Desert. A year and half into my time with the Peace Corps, I suddenly began to lose weight and grow weak. We had an embassy nurse but were too small an outpost to have a doctor. The nurse thought I might have some form of leukemia and ordered me to go to Dakar, Senegal, where an embassy doctor could see me. We set out on the seven-hour drive, but were turned back at the border by military police. There had been a coup and no one could leave the country. I returned to Nouakchott and stayed at the embassy for the next ten days. I began playing with the idea of leaving the capital and crossing the border in a more remote location. The journey would have required a canoe, a pick-up truck filled with a mix of people and goats, and enough bribe money to get through several security check points. But I was already starting to feel better and decided to stay put.

However, the nurse insisted that I go. With the coup settled and the borders open, I agree. The doctors took my blood and felt my glands. My blood count was fine, my glands normal. He said if I wanted further tests at Walter Reed, he'd be happy to send me back to the states. Or, he said, I could go back to my village. I chose my village.

Gani had a population of 300 Mauritanians and me, nestled on the banks of the Senegal River. Mud huts lined the recessing waters of the river which had endured twelve years of drought. There was no electricity, no running water, and sparse fields of grain that were picked over by the camels that frequently crossed the dry land like an armada of ships. Men sat atop them wrapped in their traditional turbans, providing protection from the blowing sands of the Sahara, revealing just their eyes. These men on their majestic camels were like the cowboys of the American West on their trusted mustangs taking cattle herds across the prairie. But instead of having Winchesters slung across their saddles, the herdsmen carried submachine guns to protect their camels and precious goods. Sand, crop-eating camels, machine gun-toting nomads—it was home to me and I was happy to be back.

I'm the Surgeon You Want

I understand why the surgeons ask so many questions about my time in Africa. Maybe I had contracted an undiagnosed disease that had returned twenty years later. My entire history is open to review. But a month has already passed since the spots were discovered and I'm more than eager for a definitive answer. I am persuaded the only way to learn more is to have brain surgery and remove a sample of tissue.

After several interviews, I choose a brain surgeon named Anderson at Columbia Presbyterian Hospital, a young guy, very cool. Like many good surgeons, he is self-important and imperious. Without a blink, he says, "I'm the one you want." I believe him. We schedule the operation for November 30, the day before my 46th birthday and a few days after Thanksgiving.

For many years, a huge part of our family's Thanksgiving celebration was a no-nonsense game of touch football—the "Turkey Bowl."

"So, can I play in the Turkey Bowl?' I asked the surgeon.

"Absolutely," he says, "Just don't hit anybody too hard."

I am especially concerned that everything be as normal as possible since I'm hosting the family dinner at my favorite Larchmont restaurant.

It's a peculiar dinner. As host, I feel in control and welcome the opportunity to show Benjamin that I'm all right. I give a welcoming toast and then my father stands to offer his own. He can't get through his first sentence without choking up. "Let's start eating," I shout, suddenly hoping for the day to end. Everyone can read my father's emotion. My perilous, but still undiagnosed, condition is the elephant in the room.

On November 30, the day of the operation, Heather has a business appointment in Pennsylvania. I'm angry she can't be with me, and angry by the painful reminder that she is so frequently unreliable and unpredictable. She was there for my MRI, but not for my surgery. All I can think to say is, "Whatever."

I take solace in the reliability of my family. I know Kathy is flying down from Boston and that my father is going to sleep over at my house the night before the operation. We'll get a car service to drive us to the hospital. The 6 a.m. pick up is a sleek, black sedan. As we roll down the West Side Highway the sun comes up over the Hudson. How many times have I made this drive? Hundreds, but today my senses are on high alert. The next time I drive this road my life will be different—I'll finally know what I'm facing. I blow on the inside of my window, the condensation forming a little canvas. With my finger, I quickly draw a smiley face and a sad face. Then, just as quickly, I wipe them away.

I remember the words of a top surgeon at Mount Sinai

Hospital as I was leaving his office: "Peter, unfortunately bad things sometimes happen to good people." It was an old cliché, but now it sounds profoundly significant.

The Day of Reckoning

At Columbia Presbyterian, I fill out the forms, deposit my clothes and lead my father into the waiting room. Kathy enters, just arrived from Boston. The nurse asks me, as required by the surgery, who I want as my Health Care Proxy, someone who would decide to keep me on life support or pull the plug if something goes horribly wrong. I choose Kathy. We had talked about how agonizing it would be as a patient to be unable to signal your intentions to your family. Each of us had pledged that if the time ever came, we would serve as proxies who would do everything possible to decipher any clues the other might offer—a blink, a twitch of the finger, anything. I trust Kathy to make the right decision. No one reads me more acutely. In many ways, she is already an extension of me.

Wearing a flimsy hospital gown, I am wheeled into surgery. Dr. Anderson is waiting for me. "We're not going to put you completely out because we need to be able to talk to you and hear you speak. Even so, you're not going to remember the operation, and you'll feel no pain, since the brain is impervious to it. We'll give you just enough anesthesia so you'll feel like you're asleep." They put a crown on my head and attach it to my skull with four screws so I'll remain perfectly still during surgery. At that moment, I have a brief out-of-body sensation, as if I were the surgeon looking down at my own head. With Dr. Anderson beside me, technicians take an MRI, my first since the initial diagnosis.

"Peter, good news," Anderson says, leaning over the table inches from my face. "The largest tumor, or whatever it was that we saw, has gotten smaller, but another one formed which is an easier spot to reach. We'll get the biopsy from that one." I don't have much time to decide whether this is good news or bad, because an anesthesiologist is now leaning over me. "Count back from ten," she says in that quiet voice all anesthesiologists seem to develop in med school. I make it to seven.

The next thing I know, I'm on a lounge chair in the recovery room, surrounded by a curtain. On the other side, I hear muffled voices. I glance to the side and see Dr. Anderson sitting beside me.

There is no small talk about how I'm feeling. "We had a pathologist in the operating room to examine the tissue," he says matter-of-factly. "It's malignant." He does not expect me to say anything and I don't. "We have a fairly good understanding of what it might be, and we'll know more in two years." He stands. "I'm going to speak to your family." He exits abruptly, like a fighter pilot turning back to base after destroying his target.

Two years? I'm sure that's what he said, though I have no idea why it would take that long to reach a clear diagnosis. Did he say two days? In any case, I fix on the idea that I have at least two years to live. I can deal with two years. At least it's not two months, or two weeks. I can breathe.

Feel the Fear, Find Your Courage

They wheel me into the double room where I'll spend the night. They can't offer me any sedatives—none are ever prescribed after brain surgery—and I wonder if I'll be able to sleep. But there's no time to worry about that now since my room is already filling up—Kathy, Dad, my stepmom Eleanor, my cousin Bill, and Heather, who (unpredictable as usual) made it back from her business trip to be with me after the surgery. Dr. Anderson is there as well, and everyone is peppering him with questions.

As if I were not present, Anderson describes my form of cancer in highly technical, academic jargon. I listen and watch from my bed, feeling suddenly alone. My heart begins beating like a snare drum. Kathy is staring at me. "Everybody out of the room," she orders. They obey, even Anderson who is still talking on his way out.

Kathy quickly puts a brown paper bag over my mouth and tells me to breathe. It smells of coffee; she must have bought a cup before she came to the room. I, too, obey her, and it calms me down. "You were about to have a panic attack," Kathy says. "You were hyperventilating."

"I've got to get a private room," I tell her. She disappears, then returns. "It's going to cost you $800."

"I don't care. It's worth it."

Looking back on my fear that day in the hospital room, I think it was an essential part of the process of recovery. The anxiety was so overpowering I really had no choice but to acknowledge it and allow it to take its course—shake me to the core, bring me to tears, race my heart. There would be more moments like this and each one helped prepare me for the long fight ahead. During those long months I began to draw inspiration from a surprising source—the Spartans of ancient Greece.

Historians regard the Spartans as among the most disciplined and feared warriors of all time. Military training began for Spartan boys at age seven. The harsh regime, which included scant food and clothing along with constant competition, was intended to inure these future warriors to hardship and to control their fears. Only then, it was thought, could they endure the horror of war and prevail.

Given the emphasis on self-denial, bravery, and discipline you might think the Spartans punished or stigmatized every manifestation of fear. In fact, they acknowledged the inevitability of fear as part of their post-battle ritual. After battle, the surviving Spartan fighters would form a line. At the front of the line the commander would suddenly begin to shake uncontrollably. Then he would cry and fall to his knees. Finally, he would lie down and ball himself up into a fetal position. Then the men would follow suit, venting all their pent-up fears and emotions in a similar fashion.

The ritual provided a space for Spartans to release the anxieties that had been suppressed during battle. They understood that fears could not be entirely eliminated. In fact, the Spartans respected fear as a necessary component of courage. The goal, however, was to train warriors to channel their emotions into fearless bravery during battle. Then, post-battle, all the bottled-up emotions could be fully and dramatically purged. By doing so, they believed, they were making themselves whole again, a process that would allow them to reset their battle-ready courage for the next fight.

As cancer patients, we are like the Spartans. We must feel the fear, let it run through our bodies. Cry, scream, shake, and let it all out because we, too, need to understand that you can't gain the courage to fight without feeling the fear. I needed to feel the fear in that hospital room to find my courage to fight.

But it would take time to make that connection. After my panic attack, I wasn't thinking about fighting; I was only thinking about getting a private room. I was glad to have it, but the extra attention also highlighted the strangeness of my situation. Here I was, just an hour or so after receiving a brain cancer diagnosis, being asked by a kind nurse: "Would you like a DVD?"

Once that would have been an easy question to answer. Of course! I'd always been a lover of movies and rarely missed an episode of favorite TV shows like "Seinfeld." At this moment, though, watching a screen was the last thing I wanted to do.

Heather announces she's staying the night and pulls a chair near my bed, covering herself with a blanket. I have no idea what day it is, what time it is, what is happening in the outside world.

I close my eyes. I remember periodic visits from nurses, the touch of Heather's hand, and the noise from the outside corridor.

When I open my eyes again the sun is shining, though I could swear I hadn't slept. Heather kisses my forehead. "Happy Birthday, Baby," she whispers. Birthday? Yes! It's December 1, 2005. Forty-six years ago I was born in another New York hospital less than a mile away. Who cares? Heather, evidently. Certainly not me.

Dachau

Dr. Anderson comes in, his lab coat pristine, his manner brisk. "We're going to release you," he says. "You're good to go. But it's not the last you'll see of me. The next step is radiation, the best way to treat a glioma. It's going to be aggressive but we have the best radiation specialists in the world."

If I had known what "glioma" meant I might have panicked. But I didn't, so I don't. I'm still clinging to the belief that Anderson thought he had at least two years to figure out my illness. "Knock yourselves out," I tell him.

"One other thing," Dr. Anderson adds. "We have a pathology grand round on the first day of every month and I'm going to present your case today. I want everyone to take a look at your slides and the pathology report so I can be sure of the diagnosis."

Heather drops me off at my home in Larchmont. Kathy is there waiting along with her fiancé, Chris, who had driven down from Boston that morning. I had known Chris since I was in junior high and he was the best friend of my older brother Alex. The three of us decide to go to the mall, not because we wanted to shop, but just to get our minds off the bleak diagnosis.

When we get back, there's a message on the machine: "Peter, this Dr. Anderson. Today at the pathology meeting we looked at your slides. A few people thought it might not be glioma. If so, that's good news. It would mean you have a less serious form of cancer. I should be able to confirm it one way or the other very soon."

An hour later, Anderson calls back. "Great news," he tells me. "We've confirmed you have B-cell lymphoma and that's something you have a much better chance to beat." I hang up and quickly share the news. Chis and I exchange high fives.

The relief of that moment came rushing back to me a few years ago when I read *Man's Search for Meaning* by Viktor Frankel, the renowned Austrian neurologist and psychiatrist who survived the Holocaust. Reading about his road to physical and spiritual survival made me wish I'd come across his book during my treatment. "We cannot avoid suffering," Frankel writes, "but we can choose how to cope with it, find meaning in it, and move forward with renewed purpose." He had an amazing ability to discover love, beauty, and even humor in the most perilous circumstances.

Frankel is also fully aware his survival was dependent not only on his own fierce determination, but on circumstances and luck. At a crucial moment during the war, he and other prisoners were sent to another camp. "We had all been afraid that our transport was heading for the Mauthausen camp" where the gas chambers would be sure to meet them. "We became more and more tense as we approached a certain bridge over the Danube which the train would have to cross to reach Mauthausen, according to experienced traveling companions. Those who have never seen anything similar cannot possibly imagine the dance of joy performed in the carriage by the prisoners when they saw that our transport was not crossing the bridge and was instead heading 'only' for Dachau." Tens of thousands of people died at Dachau, but because it was a forced labor camp rather than an extermination center, the prisoners felt relief, even joy. They might have a chance to survive after all.

For me, hearing that I had B-cell lymphoma rather than glioma, brought a similar relief. I have a chance, I thought. I have a chance.

But there was one nagging source of anxiety I didn't mention to Kathy and Chris when I got off the phone with the good news. After telling me about the revised diagnosis, Dr. Anderson said, "Oh, by the way. Have you been checked for AIDS? A high percentage of people who get B-cell lymphoma also have AIDS."

Once again, I was confronted with my decades-old terror, and once again I cast it aside: "I'm good," I tell him. "Just wanted to let you know," the surgeon added. "I mean, I'm not aware of your situation."

The next day I nervously call my former wife Nancy to tell her about the doctor's question about AIDS. "You really should get yourself tested," I advise.

"Really?!" she responds, the word sounding like an accusation.

"Listen, I don't know what could have happened to me twenty years ago. It's just a precaution."

"Thanks for telling me," Nancy says, her sarcasm so thick I could have spread it on toast. She hangs up.

I call Heather too, who is much more sympathetic. "Why don't you find out for yourself?" she asks, knowing of my fear. "I'll try," I say. "Just don't count on it." I promise myself I'll get the test, but already I know I'll put it off indefinitely. What a wimp, I think to myself. Worse—a coward, a betrayer.

When Dr. Anderson and I speak again, I don't bring up the subject of AIDS. "I'd love to keep you here with me at Columbia Presbyterian," Anderson tells me. "But to be honest, there is someone else I recommend. I was number two in my class at Johns Hopkins. There's a woman named Maria Alto who was number one. She's the world's leading authority on B-cell lymphoma. I'm going to call her and get you an appointment.

Time to Meet the General

Kathy and Heather come with me to see Dr. Alto. I wasn't fully aware then how important it was to me to have loved ones at my side for these crucial meetings. We are ushered into the doctor's office almost immediately, already a good sign. For some reason, as soon as I see her, the image of General Douglas MacArthur flashes to mind. She seems equally poised, authoritative, in command.

Dr. Alto is a very polished looking woman in her mid-forties wearing a stylishly cut red dress and a strand of pearls. Holding my folder in her lap, she initiates a brief introductory chat about the events leading up to the diagnosis. Then, without further delay, she cuts to the chase: "There are two ways we can play this. The first is traditional—a course of chemotherapy followed by full brain radiation." Then, looking at me closely, she says, "The second option is for you to consider participating in a clinical trial I'm just starting. I think you could benefit by being part of it. Unfortunately, we're about to begin it so I'll need to know your answer by tomorrow. I apologize for the short turnaround."

I don't have to think. "I'm in," I blurt. Why not? I'd almost certainly get more personal attention as part of a trial and it would be with the world's leading authority!

She smiles, self-satisfied. "Do you want to hear what the procedure is?"

"Of course." Even at this point I feel a powerful urge to please the doctor I'm already thinking of as "the General."

"The first part is conventional chemotherapy with eight cycles. You'll come to Sloan Kettering every ten days, get a heavy dose of drip chemo directly into your veins, and stay here until the chemo clears your kidneys, which should take three or four days. As you move through chemotherapy, we'll begin to collect stem cells from you're your blood to use later in the experimental trial. After the eighth cycle of chemo, if there are no signs of cancer in your brain, you'll be put in isolation for a month to keep you safe from infection. While you're in isolation, you'll undergo an even more intense course of chemotherapy and then we will re-introduce your cleaned stem cells. You should know that it will be a very difficult and exhausting treatment, but we think it will give you a better chance to beat this and keep you in remission."

I could see from their expressions that Heather and Kathy were wholeheartedly on board with the plan. My heart skipped with the most unalloyed sensation of hopefulness I had felt since my diagnosis.

"When do we start?" I ask.

Dr. Alto wants to move quickly. She schedules the first cycle of chemo for the following week, December 20, just before Christmas.

We're all a little giddy walking out of the office. Kathy and Heather immediately begin whispering about the doctor's expensive clothes and her Jimmy Choo shoes. "The shoes alone are $2, 000," one of them says.

Life Is Complicated

With treatment looming, I realize that other parts of my life are also in limbo. My company is amazingly supportive, but I still have to figure out all the nitty-gritty details of leave time and insurance coverage. I know I can count on my family, but there is still not a clear plan in place to make sure that one of my siblings will be around when I need help.

The great unknown is Heather. I have no idea what to expect from her since our relationship remains so stormy and her loyalties so divided. My problems with Heather have not gone unnoticed. Even before my diagnosis my father wrote me a letter expressing his concerns about the relationship and the negative impact he thought it was having on me.

"Peter," he wrote, "you are a tremendous person with so much to give the world and those you love and who rely on you. But you remind me of the Greek god Icarus who tempted his fate by continuing to fly too close to the sun on wings of feathers and wax." He was right when it came to Heather. I was in jeopardy not only of losing my wings but bursting into flames as I darted and danced around her alluring heat.

The Long Island Sound that separated Heather from me might as well have been the Atlantic Ocean. The expectations and priorities we grew up with were so different. For me, attending college was taken for granted; so was the assumption that I would graduate and take my rightful place in the white, male-dominated, executive workforce. Although Heather was attracted by the rewards of upward mobility, she could also cast razor-sharp aspersions on the privileged world of Westchester and Fairfield counties, and on me, a lifelong resident.

Why did we stay together, despite all the fights and separations? I think it was because we somehow believed the other person could fill in the missing parts and pockets of pain we'd suffered earlier in our lives. In my case, despite the relative economic privilege of growing up in Westport, Connecticut, in many ways my childhood lacked structure and support. My father was a serial philanderer who was charismatic and charming, but also narcissistic. All the children loved being with him. He was like the pied piper. On weekends, we all got up early because we were afraid of missing out on his adventures, even if it was just watching him do errands. But we also worried he might forget us if we were not in his immediate company.

When I was in high school one of his more flagrant infidelities was finally exposed. He and my mother divorced. Although both my parents deeply loved their five children, life in our house was always a free-for-all. There was almost complete freedom, and almost no structure. As the youngest of the five, I had the most "freedom," which meant the least oversight from my parents. Even in economic terms there was not a great deal of real security. We had a nice house, true, but we never seemed to have much money. With five kids to feed, my mother used to buy the thinnest lunch meat ever sliced. Also, although my father was a creative and gifted entrepreneur, his innovative ideas were better than his follow through. By the time Kathy and I went to college, we had no financial help and had to work our way through.

My upbringing was a bizarre mix of fun and anxiety. Both of my parents had an intense love of life and instilled it in all their children. But that was combined with a fundamental lack of structure and guidance. The result was I always wanted to find women who were strong, sexy, and exciting, but I also yearned for a sense of predictability and order I had never had. It proved to be an almost impossible combination to find.

First Day of School

Heather offers to drive me and Kathy to the hospital for my first treatment. Our route is the FDR Drive down to Sloan Kettering. It is the first day of a transit strike in New York, and since none of the subways or buses are running, FDR is at a complete standstill. Heather decides to try Second Avenue. It's as clogged as a bad artery. We're stopped cold. She announces another idea: "I'm going over to Third and loop back." As each minute passes, I'm becoming ever more frenzied. My chemo appointment is for 8:30, and Lord knows what will happen if I'm late. I bark at Heather: "Third will be just as jammed." She yells back, "It can't be worse than this!"

With traffic barely creeping I finally say, "I'm going on foot." I grab Kathy's hand and we leap out of the car. "Fuck you!"

Heather yells from the driver's window. Kathy and I jog most of the mile or so to the hospital. I could hardly be more stressed out on the brink of my first round of chemo.

As it turns out, we could have taken our time. The strike has delayed many staff and patients so we end up with a long wait. When Heather storms in, she is still angry that we left her and we pick up the fight where we left off.

Kathy intervenes. "Listen, you two." She says in a loud whisper. "Just stop it. Look where you are."

Nearby is a wide range of patients and families—women in headscarves, kids with parents, a variety of elderly people. "Yeah, all right," I assure Kathy, struggling for breath. Heather simmers. Eventually, a nurse introduces herself and leads us to the seventh floor.

There is a corridor leading to the nurse's station, and several rooms with their doors closed. It looks no different from any other floor in any other hospital, but it is, I realize, my home for three or four days out of every two weeks for the next four or five months. I'm taken to a double room, the other bed empty. I am counting on a single, but I don't have time to mention it before an army of nurses arrive like a SWAT team. They take my basic information—though it must already exist in Sloan Kettering's system—and then my blood.

One of the nurses comes in with a razor. "Pull up your shirt," she commands.

"What are you going to do?" I ask.

"I'm going to shave your chest so we can put in a port."

"What's a port?"

"A small tube we insert in your chest with a small incision so we can give you your chemo without poking a vein every time you come in."

"No way!" I protest.

"Trust me, Mr. Green, it'll make things much easier for you."

"I'm sure you're right, but I don't want my son seeing me with a tube sticking out of my chest every time I come home. I want everything to be as normal as possible. Just use my veins."

"They won't stay strong enough." She snaps, clearly annoyed.

"Please, just do it," I say. She shrugs, closes the razor with a snap, and leaves.

A young, black nurse enters, the chemo man. He smiles. "This is no longer about you," he tells me. "It's about your kidneys. After I administer the chemo, we're going to monitor your kidneys. Once the chemo clears your kidneys, you can go home."

"You mean, once I clear the poison I can go home," I say. He grins. "I see you've done your homework."

Other nurses continue to buzz around me. Kathy, well aware of my lingering fear about AIDS, seizes the moment to ask, "How did the HIV test go? We haven't heard back on it." I snapped to attention. The nurse chuckled and continued with Kathy, "Sweetie, he wouldn't be here if it was positive. That'd be a whole different world."

I was flooded with relief. It felt like I finally had a clear answer to the dreaded question. I thought, okay, now I'm ready for the worst chemo you've got. Bring it on.

I hear the clickety-clack of high heels, a sound I would soon grow to treasure. It's Dr. Alto, and her Jimmy Choo's. She's doing her rounds. Hoping for a little warm and fuzzy comforting, I quickly see she is trailed by whole squad of doctors-in-training. General MacArthur has returned. "Tonight's his first session," she explains. Turning directly to me with a kind smile, she says, "I'll be in tomorrow morning to check on you. Good luck." She turns away, followed by her ducklings.

The chemo nurse returns and sets me up. As he releases the chemo, I watch a vivid green liquid moving through the IV tube. My cousin Bill, Kathy, Heather and the nurse are all speaking to one another and seemingly oblivious to the effervescent green river entering my vein. I can't take my eyes off the poison entering my body. I know it's going to make me sick, I just don't know yet how sick. I try to comfort myself with the reminder that this attacker may well be my protector.

The drip takes two hours. My entourage chatters away beside me, but I'm silent, feeling sorry for myself. The nurse unhooks the chemo bag. "You should stand up and take a walk," he says. Bill takes my arm. "Good idea. Come on, Peter. You need the exercise." He helps me sit up. I expect dizziness, discomfort, the shakes, but feel nothing. Strange. The IV pole is still attached, and I use it as a crutch to enable me to stand. It will become my best friend and dance partner every time I come to Sloan Kettering for treatment.

Cancer Doesn't Care Who You Are

With Bill on one arm and the IV pole on the other, we begin our evening perambulation, the first of many walks around the "neighborhood" of the 7th floor. This introduction was the most memorable. We had hardly left the room before we began to observe the full range of sights and sounds on a cancer ward—a very old woman asleep with her mouth wide open in the semi-dark, alone; a mother holding the hands of two children as they walked into a room to visit a man who must be their father; a distant laugh and then, seconds later, some nearby crying. Dozens of people were struggling with cancer on a single floor, each one a complicated life story. Bill and I didn't say much as we made our rounds, but just looking at him I knew he, too, was taking in the enormous significance of what we were glimpsing—all these unimaginable stories, all these lives in danger and the larger set of lives deeply affected by their struggles.

The rooms are arranged in a circle around a nurse's station in the middle. That hub looks like a beehive loaded with computers. It's a scene that is both deeply human and overwhelmingly tech-nological. There must be a dozen computers within eyeshot and while some of the staff are pecking away at the screens orderlies and nurses move in and out of the hub in a complicated dance conveying information, small talk, everything that makes the floor function. At the receiving end of all this humming activity are the patients. And now I am one of them. At any possible moment, the hub will send someone to visit with a pill, an injection, a question, or simply because I called for help.

Closest to the nurse's station is a dimly lit room with three beds. It is the room, I later learned, for patients in the most critical condition. They are under close and constant scrutiny. I say a half prayer, half pledge that I will never be sent to that room.

By the time we get back to my room, Bill seems more tired than I am. Heather is on the phone with Kathy standing next to her. My sister has a worried expression on her face. She looks up.

"What's going on?" I ask.

"It's Benjamin," Kathy responds, handing me the phone.

I'm expecting an urgent question about how I'm doing. Instead I hear this: "It's Max! Dad, Max ran away! He's almost crying. "I'm outside in the driveway calling for Max and John's inside making a fucking cappuccino." John is Benjamin's stepfather. I had asked Nancy and John to look after my dog, Max, while I was in the hospital.

Less than a day into my first chemo treatment and already my other life—my normal life—is reaching out to pull me back. My thoughts quickly shift from the 7th floor and the green liquid swimming toward my brain to my panicky ten-year-old son whose puppy is missing and John is in the kitchen making a "fucking cappuccino."

With one call to my voicemail at home, I locate Max. Neighbors had found him in their yard. With a second call, my dog walker agrees to run by and pick up Max. From now on, she promises, she'll take care of Max when I'm in the hospital. The third call reassures Benjamin that everything is fine. It was quickly apparent that cancer wasn't going to give me a pass on my daily responsibilities. For me, of course, it was the overriding responsibility, the issue I had to resolve before I could go back to ordinary life. But, in some ways it was reassuring to discover I would still be expected to perform my duties as father, boyfriend and boss. So far, at least, I was showing that I was still strong enough to carry them out, a signal I was not losing the battle with cancer.

Sometimes You Just Have to Laugh

I still feel no effects from the chemotherapy. Bill and Heather have left, and I'm alone with Kathy, who has promised to stay the night in a fold-out chair. The other bed, I realize with a shock, is occupied. My roommate on the other side of the curtain is Norman, an older gentleman. His wife, Bertha, sits at his bedside. His doctor stands in front of them with bad news. "It's come back," he says, his voice calm. Bertha doesn't seem particularly distraught. I later learn she and her beloved Norman live with their children and grandchildren. They were immigrants who came to America and built a life they never dreamed they could have. Whatever is going to happen to Norman, Bertha comes across as a woman who can endure anything. She leans over to introduce herself. "I'll be with Norman all night—he's very sick. I sure hope he doesn't keep you awake with his snoring. He's one, loud snorer."

A bolt of panic shoots through my system. Snoring has always made me crazy. In fact, the whole Green family has a legendary intolerance for every imaginable human-made noise besides ordinary speech—heavy breathing, chewing, smacking, slurping, sniffling, snoring—it all drives us up the wall. As for me, whenever we went on family trips and I had to share a hotel room with my brothers, I would take a pillow and blanket and set up my bed in the tub so I wouldn't have to listen to all the nighttime noise. I'm now worried I'll be facing a sleepless night next to Norman.

I manage a bowl of soup for dinner, and give the rest of my meal to Kathy. When the lights eventually go out, the snoring begins. Slowly and softly at first, then it comes in an ever-rising crescendo. Within the hour Kathy and I feel as if we're living next door to a bombing range.

After a while, we make an alarming discovery—the snoring is not coming from Norman, but Bertha! Kathy and I start giggling hysterically, trying to do it as quietly as possible. What else could we do? It was either that or cry. We are in for a long night.

Not too much later I realize that Bertha's snoring is the least of my concerns. The chemo is kicking in and I'm suddenly nauseous. My body has taken notice of the toxic chemicals running through my system and is trying to get rid of them. I'm off on my first of many trips to the bathroom. I'm over the toilet with gut wrenching convulsions racking my body. Most of it is dry heaves. Bertha is still booming away in the background and Kathy is standing next to me, still trying to suppress her laughter. I, too, have tears still running down my cheeks, but not from the laughter anymore but the pain. Bertha and I are playing a John Philip Sousa duet called "Competing Tubas."

When I'm finally back in bed, Kathy rings for the nurse, who hurries in. Kathy points to Bertha and whispers, "Can you do something?"

"Sure." The nurse gives Bertha's chair a mighty kick, and the snoring stops. A soft voice comes from behind the curtain. "Thank you," Norman whispers, setting off another round of suppressed laughter, this time including the nurse. At this point I'm physically exhausted and covered in sweat. Somehow, I finally begin to doze off.

Kathy and I are awake when we hear Pearl the blood-taker making her way down the hall with her cart, her bracelets jingling as she moves in and out of the rooms dispensing good cheer. "How you doin,' sweetheart? Glad to hear it. You're lookin' swell."

She enters my room. "Hey, sweet pea, where's your port?"

Frowning back at her, I say, "I'm not going to have a port."

"What do you mean? Nobody does this without a port."

"I do."

She shrugs. "Let's take a look." She rolls up the sleeve of my hospital gown. "Make a fist." She stares. "Wow! You got the veins of a junkie." It's one of the nicest compliments I've ever received. Pearl takes my blood, deposits it in an already labeled glass vial on her cart, and departs for the next room. "Hello, sweetness. How you doin' today..."

Through the next five months, my veins manage to endure well over a hundred needles. I'm certainly not a superman, or a junkie, but the program of exercises I developed kept me as strong as possible through treatment, including my veins. I didn't learn these exercises from a physiotherapist or doctor. They're inventions of my own, based on years of workouts, and I'm convinced they greatly eased the ill effects of my treatment. They are the best antidotes to the poison of chemotherapy I can prescribe. They also gave confidence and hope to my loved ones, especially Benjamin. They could see I was doing everything possible to get better and that made them realize they didn't have to treat me like a helpless victim.

It's my fourth day in the hospital, the day before Christmas Eve. By now, I have a private room (free at last from Bertha's snoring!). Kathy is still with me, staying each night as she would through most of my chemo cycles. Heather is on Long Island with her family, continuing to lead two lives. As hard as it must be on her to juggle those competing obligations, it continues to make me angry and even when she visits me in the hospital we often bicker.

A group of carolers enter to serenade Kathy and me. Although the Greens are Jewish, we always celebrated the Christmas season, always put up a tree, and relished the extra time to spend together. It was an important expression of our family bond. When the carolers asked what song we wanted, the answer was obvious—"Little Drummer Boy." Because it had been my brother Alex's favorite when he was young, the whole family had adopted it as the ultimate symbol of Christmas. None of us knew any of the words, least of all Alex, but we all did a great "pa-rum-pa-pum pum." When the carolers launch into "Little Drummer Boy," Kathy and I cannot hold back our tears.

On their way out, the singers give me a little teddy bear. I name him "Clear," hoping he will bring me good luck in the effort to rid my brain of its dangerous spots. I still have it.

Kathy leaves on an errand, and I'm visited by, of all people, Bertha! She's in full Jewish-mother mode. Her presence is surprisingly consoling, and touching. "I know you're going to do great," she assures me, never mentioning Norman's more ominous prognosis. She's a good woman. I feel a flash of shame that Kathy and I made fun of her. She hands me a yellow "Livestrong" bracelet and I put it on. I still have that bracelet and wonder how Bertha and her family are doing. I am certain she's keeping Norman's memory alive.

A nurse comes in smiling. "You're clear," she says, meaning that enough of the chemo has left my body and I have permission to go home. Hurrah! Bertha, who's still visiting, gives me a hug.

Getting "clear" became my overriding goal every time I entered the 7th floor of Sloan Kettering. It meant the chemo had finally passed through my kidneys and I could go home for ten days. I also came to realize the patient has a role in determining how long it takes to get clear. You can speed up the process a bit by drinking a lot of water. The more you urinate, the faster you flush your system. I became the best hydrator in history, drinking a full glass of water every hour. To this day my skin never looked as good as it did during those four months of chemo treatment.

That night, at home after my first hospitalization, I enjoy the best night's sleep in weeks.

My Team

When I was allowed to go home from the hospital, Kathy would return to Boston to reunite with Chris and her three children. For the periods at home between my chemotherapy, my brother Alex would arrive from the West Coast. He and Kathy were the key members of my support team and I could not have received more or better help from top professionals. Much of their support was very practical and concrete. They helped me establish a set of routines which kept me focused on the day-to-day details of what needed to get done. That kept me from looking too far ahead and worrying too much about the future.

Alex was great at establishing a sense of normalcy during my times at home. A lawyer by trade and an artist by passion, Alex quickly became an integral part of the family. He, Benjamin, and I quickly developed a set of routines and inside jokes. We were like a little gang. The three of us even started wearing the same black knit hats when we went out into the winter cold.

With my brother around, Benjamin and I remained as calm and stable as possible under the circumstances. He and I would get Benjamin ready for school, drop him off, swing by Starbucks for coffee, and go about our day. Alex would take care of the shopping, cooking, and household chores allowing me to continue my professional life by working from home. Most of all, I made sure to make time for a daily workout. Alex has been a dedicated runner his whole life and he shares my passion for fitness. He was the perfect exercise partner.

Cancer and Work

Many people diagnosed with cancer have jobs. We might be manual labors, white collar workers, or even students. Whatever the activity, work dominates much of our lives. It not only fills our days, but has a great impact on the lives we lead with family and friends. And our workmates can become as close as family. Many of us spend more of our waking hours with fellow workers than we do with our families.

When I was diagnosed, I was a highly compensated executive for a large media company, weather.com. I managed a team of some thirty people, most of them younger than me. My work life was the opposite of my private life. At work, I was always in control, confident in the decisions I made and how to direct those I managed. Outside of work, my life was chaos in motion, mostly because of my relationship with Heather. After a few years with Heather, I no longer could count how many times we had broken up and reunited. I also was frequently entertaining thoughts about other women, and sometimes dating them.

For all the turmoil, at 6:30 a.m. on Monday through Friday I awakened for work with a sense of purpose. Often enough, work provided relief from the confusion and agitation of my private life. Because work was such an important part of my identity, I didn't want cancer become my new title: Peter Green, cancer patient. I still wanted to be Peter Green, senior vice president of sales.

However, I knew I couldn't control the workplace gossip. Undoubtedly people were talking among themselves. What do you think? Will Peter die? Is someone going to take over his role while he's in treatment? Have you noticed a difference in his work?

I was asking the same questions myself. Cancer doesn't care what anyone says or thinks, which means you can either think that "cancer victim" is your entire identity, or a problem you're dealing with as you move on with your life. I chose the latter. After the initial shock of my diagnosis, my company and I realized work had to proceed. Meetings had to take place, revenue goals had to be met, and the normal cadence of the workday had to continue. I was determined to remain an important part of that work.

I also realized that if I stepped back and took a leave from work, my position might be at risk. I had one of the most coveted roles in our intensely competitive industry. There would always be a pack of alpha dogs ready to storm in and take my place at the first sign of weakness. I had relished the competition throughout my career and was not about to give ground now. The first priority was to make clear to my team that I was still in charge, still able to manage their work, provide them support, and, most importantly, help them make money. I wasn't going to make it easy for anyone to drive me out.

Home from the hospital, I spent hours on the phone speaking with my team. Sales projections were formulated, prospective deals debated, assignments designated, training workshops planned. When the calls leaked into the early evening, Alex would calmly walk over to the couch, take the phone from my hand, and say, "Sorry to interrupt, but this is Alex, Peter's brother, and he needs to rest now." If he hadn't done that, I would still be talking. I feared if I didn't keep up the same intensity, my colleagues—some of them close friends—would sense my weakness and pounce. It was the corporate culture I knew and accepted, and one that had benefitted me in many ways. Yet during these months, I also began to question its core values more profoundly that I ever had before, particularly its focus on individual gain.

In some ways, I think cancer actually helped me be a better sales executive. It helped me cut through a lot of the bullshit that often delays or muddies important decisions. I developed a much more powerful determination to make efficient use of time. Actions should not be rushed, but I was not nearly so tolerant of needless discussion or gossip. I found myself asking pointed questions about projects and people. In the past, I would have been less decisive. I became bolder in moving forward with risky opportunities that had the potential for greater rewards. If those risks failed, I was willing to admit my error and seek to correct it. I also found myself listening harder to the ideas of others. I became less concerned about colleagues who might want to take my place and even gave them further responsibilities knowing it was right for the company.

With my life in peril, I became more acutely aware of how petty and personal business could be, how much of a "ME" culture it fostered. Though it was rarely admitted, many people in business are constantly asking, how will this decision affect ME? How does it make ME look? Will it position ME for a promotion? Will the added revenue come to ME? If it fails, what happens to ME?

Fighting cancer put everything in perspective. I was no longer so interested in the personal impact of day-to-day business. I was better able to see the big picture—if we worked for the success of the company it would be good for all of us. I was better able to cut through the ME factor and all the corporate posturing that accompanied it.

As I went back and forth for my chemo treatments, I was constantly aware of the many other patients on the cancer ward. It was especially humbling to see all the children struggling with the disease. Their fight, as much as my own, shaped my new attitude toward work. When my associates began to argue, or complain, or act as if the entire world would collapse if we didn't make our quarterly sales goal, I began to say, "Listen, no one is dying here."

To myself, I would often put my work pressures in perspective by saying, "Peter, this is nothing. You're fighting brain cancer and for now you are winning. Can anyone in this room say the same thing? Have they seen the kids at Sloan Kettering and all the staff and doctors dealing with life-and-death problems?" Just remember, "No one is dying here."

Executives, if you're reading this book, recognize that if you have employees who are going through cancer treatment, or have returned from it, you may well have someone who will now do an even better job, who may have an enhanced ability to focus on the major priorities of what's best for the company. Consider these employees a valuable resource and take an active part in discussing how they might stay connected to work during their treatment. It not only will benefit your employee, it also will enhance the culture and spirit of the entire company.

You're Clear—Maybe

After my fifth cycle of chemotherapy they give me an MRI to see what, if any, progress has been made. I'm lying on my bed and hear all this commotion outside my room. All of a sudden, someone from Dr. Alto's team comes in and says, "Peter, Dr. A just texted us—Great news, your MRI is clean!" No one expected such dramatic success so early on in the treatment.

A little later that morning Dr. Alto comes to my room and confirms the news. "But Peter, there may be a hitch. One of the pathologists thinks he sees a small speck. I don't see it, but maybe it's just a case of wish fulfillment." Dr. A is eager for me to participate in her stem cell replacement trial and for that to happen I have to have a completely clean scan. "In any case, I'm confident enough to take you into the trial right now if we can get another scan to confirm these results. If it does, you have a big decision to make. Do you want to go into isolation now and begin the new course of chemo followed by the stem cell replacement, or do you want to finish the last three cycles of this treatment first?"

Her tone gives no indication of what route she hopes I take, but I sense she wants to be absolutely sure I'm clean before starting the trial. I say, "Yeah, let's finish the final three. Let's make sure we knock this thing out."

"Good," she says. I take satisfaction in the thought I have pleased the General.

Samantha–Finding Romance When You Least Expect It

My decision to return to the 7th floor three more times isn't just to please Dr. A. Since my first round of chemo I had been attracted to the head nurse, Samantha. During the first five rounds we had become friendly. I learned her family had come from Nicaragua in the 1980s, that her mother was a Seventh-day Adventist, and she lived on Staten Island with her boyfriend, an accountant. Hospital rules forbade any fraternization between nurses and patients, but Samantha and I were beginning to test the boundaries of those rules as we shared more and more about our lives and the fact we were unhappy in our current relationships.

To complicate matters, Heather sensed my growing affection for Samantha. So now, when Heather visited, she always staked out her position sitting next to me on the bed. But our fighting continued and it was clear Heather still had a strong bond with her husband. That became dramatically evident during my fourth cycle of chemo. At 11:00 p.m. one night, the day after another major blow-up, I had just fallen asleep when I feel a body slide into bed next to me. It's Heather! She spends the night. But as soon as the sun comes up she packs up to leave. Her husband is just across the street at Cornell Medical Center recovering from back surgery. Heather now is going to visit him!

Later that day Heather comes back and I once again try to

break off the relationship. "Listen," I said, "I don't want you coming to the hospital any more. It's too stressful for both of us."

Heather is no dummy. "It's that head nurse, isn't it? I know she likes you."

"Whatever," I say, coldly and dishonorably.

Heather leaves, furious. Kathy and my brother Alex are aware of my growing feelings for Samantha. She had made it a practice to come into my room at the end of her shift to say goodbye and Kathy picked up the vibe early on. This time, when Samantha comes in to say goodnight, I ask Kathy for some privacy.

"Do me a favor," I say to Samantha. "Take the picture of my dog Dallas from my nightstand and write your telephone number on the back of it." The picture is one of two I have with me. The other is of Benjamin and me. Samantha scribbles her number and hands the picture back. "You know I can't see you until you're off the floor." In other words, I conclude, she's saying thanks but no thanks. After all, I'm forty-six, she's just twenty-six. Why would she want to go out with me?

When Kathy comes back, she's more positive. "What Samantha said isn't negative. She's just not allowed to date people who are patients. But I think she likes you."

I'm cleared the next day, a Friday. On Saturday morning, I'm in my kitchen when I get a ping from Sloan Kettering. I suppose they want to schedule my next cycle, so I open the message: "Hi, it's Samantha. I don't have my home computer with me, so I'm writing this from Sloan Kettering. If you want to go out with me, I'm available Wednesday." I e-mail her back. "Let's meet at the Museum of Natural History. Three o'clock."

Alex has been staying with me, and I turn to him for a big favor. Because of the treatments, I'm not allowed to drive anywhere except near my house. "Can you take me?" He agrees to be my wingman.

Usually, after I've been cleared, I go home and fall onto my couch, exhausted, unable to do much more than watch television and go to the bathroom for the next twelve to eighteen hours. Eventually, I will myself off the couch and into my exercise routine. Dropping to the floor, I do my snow angel stretch. I can feel my blood flowing through my system and try to envision the cancer cells dying off one by one. With my body and mind working as one, a combination of movement and visualization, I can feel myself growing stronger.

Having a date to look forward to intensifies my commitment. Alex drives me to the museum. Alex, the artist, can happily spend hours looking at paintings, so he decides to head off to the Guggenheim. "I'm not sure when I'll call, Al. I don't know how this will go. It could be one hour, or it might be six."

"No problem," he responds. "Whatever you want."

There's Samantha, a little breathless, dressed in dark, slender pants and V-neck sweater. In her civilian clothes, there's no hint of the hospital nurse. Wow, I think, what a beautiful woman. We stand awkwardly for a while and decide to take a walk in Central Park rather than go to the museum. Our talk is strained, impersonal. I was almost always comfortable on first dates, but now I'm like a middle schooler at his first dance. I remember a scene in *Annie Hall* when Woody Allen walks Diane Keaton out of a movie house and I use his line on Samantha: "Let me just kiss you now; it'll get the tension over with." It works. We kiss, I'm smitten.

We go to dinner, relaxed now, enjoying each other. I don't remember the name of the restaurant or the menu. I do remember thinking the place wasn't good enough for Samantha. She deserved The Four Seasons. Well, next time. The phone rings. I look at my watch. Oops, it's already 11:00 p.m. It's Alex sounding a little miffed.

"Are you coming home tonight?"

"Of course. What else would I be doing?"

He lets the answer hang. "May I join you for coffee?" Samantha agrees, and the three of us spend a lively hour before Alex drives me home. My head is free of all thoughts of cancer. It is full of life.

That weekend, Samantha meets me at my dad's house in Westport, and soon after that I go to her home in Brooklyn where I meet her mother Sylvia, an old-fashioned woman, sweet and solicitous to me, but also protective of her beloved daughter. When Samantha is out of the room she whispers, "Take care of my angel. Promise me you won't hurt her." I promise.

Samantha moves into my Larchmont house two weeks later. It means Alex no longer has to fly in from California and Kathy comes less often. I am in the capable hands of an excellent nurse. As with so many nurses, she oozes caring and love. Benjamin immediately becomes attached to her. Her schedule—two long days on, three days off—enables her to drive him to school and pick him up on days she is free. "Remember," she advises me, "we can't tell anyone on the floor." Even Samantha can't keep that pledge for more than a week.

On one of her off days, Samantha accompanies me to a meeting with Dr. Alto, who had met Heather but doesn't seem surprised by Samantha's presence. She smiles and shakes her head. She has clearly heard about our relationship. Not much slips by the General.

Synchronicity

By late February, six cycles into my chemo, I'm gaining confidence about my health and my strength. And now, with Samantha in my life, I'm beginning to think about the prospects of life without cancer. Lying in the bed on the 7th floor of Sloan Kettering I can feel the warmth of the late winter sun shining through the window onto my face.

I find myself thinking more about religion. It's almost inevitable when you face an existential crisis like cancer. Although I've never been an observant Jew, or a follower of any other religion,

I do have a kind of spiritual faith that is helping me through these months, a faith based on the mysterious interconnectedness of human energy. By that I mean, not just the energy each of us draws on to physically get through the day, but the much more powerful energy that draws us together, so strongly we often are oblivious to it. I'm especially curious about the forms energy can take, which sometimes can be mysterious and even magical. On special occasions, I'm convinced, we can tap into the energy of people who are no longer with us. When I'm doing my exercise routine, I try to tap into this larger field of energy. The exercises described at the end of this book are meant to be as meditative as they are physical, a means to help the recovery of your mind and spirit as much as your body.

During my treatment, I had an amazing experience unlike any in my life. The best way to understand it, for me, is to draw on Carl Jung's idea of "synchronicity." According to the famous psychiatrist and psychoanalyst, synchronicity refers to meaningful connections between physical and spiritual phenomena that seem to happen by accident or coincidence (one does not directly cause the other). Jung believed people should pay attention to these apparently unrelated phenomena; they might be a way to understand an underlying unity between the conscious and the unconscious worlds.

Martha Beck, author of "How to Tell When the Universe is Sending You Signs," draws on Jung to suggest we should take the time to evaluate the important events in our lives for which there is no clear or rational explanation. "Maybe you'll consider the possibility that you could be connected to everything in the universe, and everything in the universe could be connected to you, and meaning flows between the two in a mysterious constant stream."

My most extraordinary experience of synchronicity occurred during treatment, a moment of connection with my stepsister Ann. She had died twenty years earlier.

Westport, Connecticut, September 1985

AIDS in 1985 is sweeping the world. The level of fear is palpable. The medical community is desperately trying to find ways to slow the spread of the disease and to educate the public about how to avoid infection. In October, Rock Hudson is the first celebrity to die of AIDS, one of 6,854 American victims of the disease that year.

I'm stepping off the jet at JFK airport, just home from Mauritania. The last thing I expect is to be greeted by AIDS so quickly and directly.

My stepsister, Ann Craig, is a beautiful, brilliant life force, one of the most creative and adventurous people I've ever known. After graduating from Brown University in the early '70s, she travelled extensively in Africa. The details of what she did there remain a mystery, but we do know she participated in a variety of mind-altering native rituals. When she returned home, she developed a severe case of anorexia and was in and out of hospitals and treatment centers for years.

In the early 1980s, Ann moved to New York City to pursue her long-standing interest in art and entertainment. She became a kind of underground celebrity as an emcee at the Pyramid, one of the hippest avant-garde clubs on the Lower East Side. As host, Ann gave legendary monologues and introduced a wild assortment of performance artists, drag queens, and campy satires. A regular at the club, and a friend of Ann's, was the painter Jean-Michel Basquiat, whose international fame came well after his 1987 death, at age 27, of a heroin overdose (in 2017, one of his paintings sold for $110 million).

Ann was at the center of one of the most exciting art scenes in the world and she, like many others, was unable to survive it. Like

Basquiat, she became addicted to heroin. She died a year earlier, in 1986, not from an overdose, but from the AIDS she contracted from an infected needle.

I had always seen Ann as a bigger than life individual—exotic, fascinating, charismatic, but underneath it all, very fragile and vulnerable. She was the first family member I saw when I returned from the Peace Corps in 1985. I came home to my father's empty house. Everyone was away and I had two days alone, a welcome opportunity to reacclimate to a world with running water, flush toilets, and electricity.

Finally, late on the second day, I hear a car turn into the gravel driveway. Excited, I rush outside. As the car pulls up I see it holds three people.

All three seemed to be wearing dark eyeliner, nose studs, and tattoos. Ann is sitting in the passenger seat, asleep or unconscious. She is no more than 90 pounds, her body emaciated, her mouth open, and her veins pulsating under paper-thin skin. Her two companions also are clearly heroin addicts with track marks lining their arms. When I open Ann's door, she opens her eyes and they flutter with a slight sign of recognition. She looks in desperate need of help. In the background, her friends are making fast-paced introductions and explaining they needed to bring Ann home.

I see some blood running from wounds on her arms and legs. As bad as she looks, my Peace Corps experience keeps me calm— I'd seen many people who were suffering from extreme malnutrition with the same hollow eyes I'm looking at now.

"Ann, it's Peter. Let's get you inside," I say as I pick her up and carry her into the house. In an upstairs bedroom, I placed her down on the bed that would become the last bed she would lay in.

Over the next few months, I really came to know Ann. She never went back to the city, but often the city came to her. Friends would arrive, always carrying drugs, and Ann would try to rally whatever energy she had to join their party. Although her body was steadily breaking down, she would lay on a heavy coat of black eye shadow, deck herself out in one of her flamboyant dresses and masses of bracelets, and put her fragile feet into high heels. Off they would go, sometimes just across the street to the Westport beach. Although people stared, and moved away, Ann was still the consummate master of ceremonies and still commanded her stage.

Strangers were not the only ones who shied away at the sight of Ann. Even family members were nervous being too close to her at the height of the AIDS epidemic.

Living in the same house together, as I tried to figure out my next step in life, I was around Ann almost every day. I was comfortable with her, but cautious. With good reason. Given Ann's physical decay, it was not uncommon for her to develop bleeding sores. I would sometimes find drops of blood on the floor or even in the refrigerator, unknowingly spilled by Ann as she made middle of the night trips to the kitchen or bathroom seeking some peace.

We spent many hours together talking, sharing our stories from Africa, sometimes smoking hash together from separate pipes. Other times I would read poems to her, including ones she had written. Or we'd just listen to some music and joke around. Alone together in the house, my stepsister and I became as close as blood relatives. I vividly recall my complex mix of feelings from those days with Ann. In part, there was the overwhelming pleasure that sometimes comes when you're getting to know and care deeply about someone. Yet there also was the overpowering sadness that came with knowing it would all soon end, that Ann was living with a death sentence.

I watched her take her last breath, surrounded by family. A single tear rolled down her cheek.

Almost exactly twenty years later she would come back to me.

Ann–Sloan Kettering, 7th Floor, 2006

Lying there with the warmth of the sun on my face I might be asleep, I might be dreaming, but what I see is much more vivid than any dream. First, I see myself on a small island sitting peacefully under a tree, looking out over the water. Then I am once again inside my body looking outward from the island. Across the water, not more than a hundred yards away, is a much larger land mass. It is vast and apparently empty.

Suddenly, I notice movement on the other side, a large group of ghost-like figures slowly advancing toward the water's edge, hundreds of them. Expressionless, they stare at me from the other side. I feel more curiosity than fear. Who are they? What do they want? A small commotion starts from the back of the crowd. Someone is moving to the front. The crowd parts and the advancing figure finally reveals herself: it's Ann.

Reaching the front of the crowd, she walks alone into the water toward my island. As she walks, the water rises no farther than her ankles. I continue to sit under the tree, not sure if I can even move, but feeling no need to do so. As Ann approaches I see she is wearing none of her over-the-top make-up or clothes. Her appearance is simple, clean, and calm. She comes so close we could have whispered to one another. She raises one arm straight out at me with her palm facing forward, an unmistakable sign to stay in my place. She holds the pose for several seconds. Then she calmly turns around and walks across the water back to the other shore to the mass of shadowy figures still standing there. Arriving on the other side, she stretches her arms outward as if trying to draw the entire group together. They turn on her signal and all of them begin to withdraw to the interior of their vast land. Soon all of them disappear, Ann among them.

I can't remember how I returned to ordinary consciousness, whether I woke up or the vision simply ended. I was lying in bed again feeling the warmth of the sun on my face. I didn't mention what I had experienced to anyone. It felt like it was an entirely private exchange between me and Ann. However, I believed from that day on, I had received a clear and powerful message: it's not my time, hold on, stay alive.

The next day I was allowed to go home. Alex and I decide to clean out a large drawer under my stove that was stuffed with old grocery bags. It is so packed it has become difficult to open and close. After pitching the bags, I get to the bottom of the drawer and find a plastic zip-lock sandwich bag. It seems to be holding some objects wrapped in tissue paper. I have no idea what they are.

I put the bag on the kitchen table and sit down to open it up. There is clearly something inside the tissue paper. As I pull away the wrapping, I immediately recognize the long-forgotten objects: three tiny clay figures that Ann had given me twenty years ago. She had brought them back from Africa in the early 1970s. The synchronicity of this discover on the heels of my vision confirm my conviction: it's not my time to join Ann on the other side of the water.

Saying Goodbye

During my eighth round of chemo, I had not spoken to Heather for more than a month. Then, out of the blue, she calls me at the hospital and immediately says: "Just tell me one thing: Are you with Samantha?"

"I am."

She pauses. "Okay, do you love her?"

"I think I do."

"Then I need you to answer one more question: Do you still love me?"

I feel a sharp stab in my gut. "No."

"You don't?"

"No."

"Okay," she whispers. The sound of her defeated voice sears me with guilt.

She hangs up and I fall asleep. When I wake up, Heather is standing at the end of my bed. It's St. Patrick's Day—March 17—and she's come to New York with her family. I can't imagine how she manages to get away from them to come to the hospital.

"I just needed to look at you and have you tell me to my face what feelings you have for me," she says.

I say, "I don't love you anymore." My voice wavers slightly.

She stands there and then finally sits beside me on the bed. "At least give me a hug good-bye."

Part of me thinks she'd just as soon kill me. With a handful of tubes connected to me I'm a little nervous about getting close to her—she just might rip them out. But I stand and we warmly embrace. She leaves without a word; it's over. I can't separate my mixed feelings: regret, shame, relief.

At long last, the eight cycles of chemotherapy come to an end. I feel surprisingly strong thanks to the exercise routine I had maintained throughout the treatment and the lift I am getting from my still young romance with Samantha.

Now, I am preparing to enter the experimental phase of Dr. A's trial—a month-long period of isolation with even more intensive chemotherapy and stem cell replacement. In preparation for this phase, technicians had plunged two long needles into my arms to draw blood into a cell separator machine. Somehow this high-tech instrument could spin out and collect healthy stem cells that would be re-injected during the second stage of the trial.

In anticipation of the isolation phase I begin to worry about the new round of chemo. I asked my old friend, the chemo nurse, "How bad is it?"

"Put it this way," he says, evidently enjoying himself. "What we've been giving you so far is candy compared to what you're going to get."

That was a terrifying thought. After all, the "candy" I had been given made me sicker than the worst bouts of flu I'd ever had—whole days of vomiting, sweats, and chills. How much worse could it be than that?

I was getting the impression I would have to endure two weeks of utter hell in which I would feel so bad I would question whether I even wanted to go on living. My white blood cell count would sink so low I would, in fact, approach the edge of death. But during the next two weeks, my harvested stem cells would be returned to my blood. If everything worked according to plan, the healthy cells would adhere to one another and build a new, cancer free ecosystem. I would gradually regain my strength.

Because I was to be in isolation, they would provide a computer for me to Skype with Benjamin and other loved ones. No one except medical personnel would be allowed in the room. Samantha had arranged to take off a month so she could be with me. As a nurse, she would have permission. I've rented her an apartment not far from Sloan Kettering so she can go back and forth.

Déjà Vu

No one is cured of cancer but when no signs of it appear, it is said to have gone into remission; and one hopes it stays that way. A well-respected oncologist once said to me, "Most people have cancer. If we gave everyone the same tests we gave you we'd find it in practically everyone." He went on: "The difference is that cancer doesn't reveal itself to everyone. It doesn't always spread rapidly enough to get detected. And then this: "Unfortunately, bad things can happen to good people." It was the second time I had heard those words.

One of those bad things happened to me again. I was set to start the one-month isolation period. I felt like a Spartan warrior. The three months of mind and body exercises has prepared me well. But first I had to have one more MRI to make sure the chemo had eliminated all signs of cancer. I was confident this test was just a formality.

When Dr. A walks into the room where Samantha, Kathy and I are waiting, I can tell from her glum expression the news is bad.

"Peter, I'm afraid we found a small speck on the scan. I'm surprised, but because of this result we can't allow you to go on with the trial. As you know, everyone who enters isolation has to be in full remission."

I'm devastated, and sense she, too, is very disappointed. I had been a model patient and now she is losing a member of what has to be a pretty small pool of test subjects.

"But, Dr.," I protest. "If it's just a speck, why can't we go ahead? Let's just blast it out with the treatment in isolation."

"I'm sorry Peter, that's impossible. This is a clinical trial and everyone has to enter it in the same condition. If we allowed you to join, it might work for you, but it would taint the results of the study."

Once again, my body reacts instantly to the hard news. My heart races, my body goes numb, and I'm bathed in sweat. I'm having another panic attack and begin to cry. At this moment, one of my lowest, I fully manifest the fear I might die.

Kathy and Dr. A's assistant get me on the examining table and have me lie down on my side. I'm sweating so much they begin to swab me down with paper towels. Dr. A tries to reassure me.

"Listen Peter, there are still plenty of things we can do. Just because you're not going on with the trial does not mean you can't get through this successfully. We'll just move ahead with the conventional approach that has worked for many people. We're going to follow your chemo with a course of radiation and I have a lot of confidence that it will take care of any remaining specks.

But even as she's saying this I'm thinking, "yeah, but how about all the other brain cells radiation will kill."

The storm of emotion passes and I begin to absorb the new reality. I had been preparing my mind and body for more chemo in isolation and now I have to gear up for radiation. As the fear subsides, I feel a bit like a Spartan warrior who has just completed his post-battle ritual. After curling up in the fetal position and venting all my pent-up emotion, I am already starting to gird myself for the next battle. On my way out of the office, Dr. A, for the first time, gives me a big hug.

I always find myself back on my living room floor, arms extended over my head and breathing deeply. Then the slow, steady routine with the weight ball and the resistance bands. Once again, I need to muster the physical and mental strength that will give me the confidence I can do this. I must do this.

The Burn

I will now complete the typical treatment for B-cell lymphoma. The day after I am dropped from the clinical trial, I am fitted for a radiation mask and have my brain mapped so the radiation guns can be as accurate as possible. They want to limit as much collateral damage as possible. For the next five weeks, I am scheduled to have radiation five times a week, a total of twenty-five treatments. I would find this phase even more humbling than the chemo.

They bring me in for the first session, lay me down on a table and bolt my head down to make sure it remains completely still. Then they bring these big radiation guns up on both sides and put them up against both of my temples. A three-foot thick lead door stands between me and the technicians who are in a booth looking at me through thick glass. Then they give me a sixty-second blast of radiation, one side at a time. I can actually hear a sizzling sound emanating from my brain. It's all over in two minutes. They bring me slowly to a sitting position, see how I'm doing, and send me on my way.

Although it was, in some ways, a much easier routine than chemotherapy with its endless sick days in the hospital, the radiation freaked me out a lot more. I always thought the vile green chemicals were only making me temporarily sick as they went about their business of destroying the cancer. But with those big guns aimed directly at my head and creating all those unnerving zinging and zapping noises, I couldn't help but think I was losing a lot more than cancer cells. This may really fuck me up.

Yet, I still tried to stay as positive as possible. One thing the radiologist said that helped a lot came in response to my great disappointment of being excluded from the clinical trial. He said, "Listen, Peter, we don't know if that trial is better than this. I mean, that trial is very dangerous. There's a chance you could have died from the treatment itself. We know what we're doing here and it has worked many times."

It also made me feel better to develop a relationship with the doctors and their teams. The radiologist and I often joked about my hair. At our first meeting, when he walked me through the process he mentioned I would lose my hair. Like all the men in my family, I prided myself on having a thick, full head of dark hair. My father, Paul, didn't even begin to turn gray until he was in his seventies.

"No way," I respond. "I'm not gonna lose my hair. I made it all the way through chemo without losing any, so I think I'm good." I was half joking, but only half.

The radiologist smiled and said, "Alright." He was probably thinking, "I've never seen it before, but knock yourself out."

During the third week of radiation, as I took my morning shower, large chunks of hair came off in my hands. Compared to everything else I had endured, it may seem like a small thing, but it had a powerful symbolic meaning. It felt like I was losing the last vestige of my pre-cancer self. I'm such a competitive person, I had wanted to be the completely exceptional patient who would sail through treatment without missing a beat. In the shower, I thought to myself, "Now I'm like every other cancer patient." It was humbling.

Later that morning, before my radiation, I go into this little local barber shop around the corner from my house in Larchmont. All the old barbers there have known me for years. I sit in the chair and tell the guy, "Just take it all."

He doesn't know what to say, but clearly understands what's happening. So he quietly shaves my head and I get up to leave. On my way out, I stand at the register and reach for my wallet. He says, "This one's on me, Peter."

The final two weeks of radiation are brutal. It really starts to sap my energy and even my spirit. By then I had burn marks up and down both sides of my head and face, caused by the radiation burning me from the inside out.

Even so, I still did my exercises and stayed committed to drinking massive amounts of water and two whey powder health shakes every day. That daily discipline helped me avoid lapsing into self-pity and depression, even during the toughest times.

Five weeks later I undergo my first post radiation MRI. I'm nervous but prepared. I trust the therapy did its job—just as I had done mine—and I'm ready to accept whatever comes next.

Back to the World

After the MRI, while awaiting the results, I follow the same routine I had begun with Heather, a Catholic. We would go to the Church of St. Catherine of Siena near Sloan Kettering. This time I'm with Samantha, but I'm a believer in ritual and routine. So we go over to the same church, light a candle, sit for a while in the pews and say some silent prayers.

This time Dr. A enters the room with a big smile. "Peter! The MRI is completely clean. Not a single speck." The relief is that rare type that feels as if a two hundred-pound weight has been lifted from my shoulders. More than that, I feel as if my mind has suddenly relaxed and opened. I had been so single-minded in my struggle there had been little room to think about anything other than cancer treatment, my effort to stay fit and healthy, and everything I had to do to manage my work and family duties. Now I allow myself to believe I might actually have a long life ahead of me. For the moment at least, anything seems possible.

Along with that renewed sense of freedom comes a sense of responsibility. I am now, officially, a cancer survivor and I know I have to do something with the knowledge I acquired. I know the intense experiences of the last eight months are not just going to disappear down the memory hole.

When I arrive home after the good news, I don't even make it upstairs. I walk into the first-floor guest room and crash on the bed. I am completely spent. Now, at last, it seems okay to rest. I felt like a runner who has just finished a marathon and collapses at the finish line.

For a week, I do almost nothing. I don't even exercise. I need to let my system regenerate itself. I'm a survivor now, not a patient. All the emotion, energy, and focus I drew on to fight cancer now will have to find new directions. And some of them I can happily do without.

March 2007–Life Moves On

By early 2007, Samantha and I had gone our separate ways and Heather is permanently out of my life. One day, visiting my father in Westport he says, "Peter, there's is a pretty young woman who just started working at the club. I think you'd like her." He worked out at the Saugatuck Rowing Club almost every day and knew all the staff and most of the members. He was also my most reliable matchmaker, having a keen sense for the kind of women who attract me.

"Have you mentioned me to her?" I ask.

He closes his eyes and nods slowly, his trademark way of saying "of course."

"And she's open to meeting you. You should stop by."

The next time in town we go to the rowing club and there at the front desk is a tall, beautiful, blond woman. I know it must be Mary. Since I'm with my father, she knows it's me and signals us to wait until she can get off the phone. I introduce myself but before we can talk I have to take an urgent business call. I complete it in the lobby of the club within earshot of Mary. She later tells me she was impressed with how I handled the call and that secured the first date.

A few days later, after this brief introduction, Dad asked Mary what she thought. The signal was encouraging enough to lead me to invite her to a play at the Westport Country Playhouse followed by a late dinner. I'd heard nothing about the play so assured her that if she didn't like it we could leave. All went well, including the dinner, though our conversation never went much beyond a bit of family and work history and the rowing club scene. Nor did it lead to a goodnight kiss.

I ask her to dinner a week later at one of my favorite restaurants in New York's meatpacking district. The conversation comes more easily this time and goes much deeper. I believe it's time to tell Mary about my bout with cancer. I need to know if that would be enough to frighten her off.

"Mary," I say a short time after the drinks arrive, "there's something important I need to tell you."

"What's that?" she asks with a raised eyebrow.

"I recently completed six months of treatment for brain cancer." As I brace for a response of deep concern, Mary blurts out, "Really? I had cancer too!"

"No way," I reply. "What are the odds?" We share our cancer stories and by the end of the evening I begin to feel as if we are meant for one another.

But it soon becomes clear that convincing Mary is going to be harder than I had imagined. She tells me that she is dating other people and doesn't intend to stop. And there is still no goodnight kiss.

I am not willing to take the risk of getting hurt so, after the third date, I call her up and say, "I think we should just be friends."

"Really?" she asks. "Okay," she agrees, but I catch a hint of doubt in her voice.

About three months later we find ourselves together at a July Fourth beach party. By then she has apparently dismissed the several suitors she had been dating. That night, for the first time, we kiss. A little over a year later, we get married.

Mary is a no-nonsense beauty from the Midwest who always says it as she sees it. She can be brutally frank, and I quickly came to admire her honesty, painful as it could sometimes, especially when she confronted me with unpleasant truths about my behavior. She was particularly concerned about my parenting of Benjamin. On one hand, she observed, I often put my own needs ahead of what was best for Benjamin. Then, perhaps out of guilt for letting him down, I would be over-indulgent, too quick to offer Benjamin money or to get him out of a jam. Mary helped me see I needed to provide more consistent guidance along with the space for him to figure things out on his own.

Early in our marriage, Mary also was critical of my reliance on my sister Kathy, who she sometimes referred to as my "mother." It was, in many ways, an accurate observation. I call Kathy almost every day (or she calls me) and we do indeed rely on each other for support. To Mary, that felt as if I valued Kathy more than my own wife. During the years I've managed to demonstrate to Mary that she truly is the number one person in my life and she now believes it. Just recently she said, "You finally see me before your sister!"

For the first time in my life I found someone with whom I can be completely honest. Part of the reason is I totally trust Mary will continue to love me even knowing my imperfections and weaknesses. I also know if I were not honest with her, I would jeopardize the best relationship of my life.

Mary knows about Heather and Samantha and that knowledge has helped us avoid some of the problems that plagued my earlier relationships. A few years after finally splitting up with Heather for good, I learned she went back to her husband permanently and they have a young son. I'm very happy for her and believe she is a wonderful mother. As for Samantha, I truly saw her as an angel sent to help me through my treatment, but our relationship did not have a strong enough foundation to endure. Perhaps the gap in our ages was too great, or the differences in our backgrounds; or maybe we simply couldn't maintain the intensity of feeling we experienced during my treatment.

While Samantha and I were together, she often told me how much she wanted to visit Seattle where I had once lived. About a year after we broke up, she sent me a text: "Peter, hope you are well. I finally made it to Seattle and it's all I thought it would be. I love it." A smile crossed my face; my cancer angel deserves all the happiness the world can give her.

Benjamin, 2016

None of us make it through life without scars, whether they come from cancer, divorce, economic hardship, a family loss, you name it. Benjamin also has been confronted with his own struggles, one of which continues to the present.

A few years ago, after spending a weekend with his grandparents, Benjamin discovered a tick on his leg and started to complain about fatigue and lethargy. He saw his doctor and was diagnosed with mononucleosis, but the symptoms lasted far beyond mono's typical duration. His mom and I felt he was exaggerating his condition. Benjamin had a history of crying wolf so we just told him to eat a better diet and get more sleep.

We did have him tested for Lyme disease but the result was negative. However, Benjamin was convinced he had Lyme and he put all his ample resourcefulness and persistence into getting an answer he could trust. He researched and found doctors who specialized in Lyme and got further tests. All the tests were negative. Eventually, Benjamin found a program at Columbia Presbyterian Hospital that confirmed he had Lyme disease despite the fact the standard test results still were negative. He began intravenous treatments to help his body and mind overcome the wide range of symptoms. Although he is still dealing with some long-term effects of the disease, he is doing much better and just finished his first year at a large university in the Midwest. We speak almost every day.

Benjamin is starting to find his own path. He is facing his fears and gaining the ability to take ownership of his medical realities in ways that allow him to adjust to difficult circumstances and even to flourish. The young man who came into the world screaming in protest has begun to find a more secure and confident identity.

Today

Who am I today? In many ways, I have finally regained the sense of purpose I felt eleven years ago during my cancer treatment. I am finally acting on the pledge I made the day I heard that my post-radiation MRI was clean; the conviction that my experience had given me the responsibility to share what I had learned from the experience of surviving cancer. It was a long time coming. Almost immediately after my treatment in 2006, I stepped back into my old patterns and pretty effectively buried the most valuable lessons and memories from my months of treatment. Although Mary's presence in my life had made me far happier than I'd ever been, and a better person in some respects, in many ways I had lost the strong convictions that had developed during my months of chemotherapy and radiation.

But the world of cancer, and all the emotions and ambitions it had stirred in me, came rushing back when my cousin John was diagnosed with cancer. On October 31, 2016, I visited John at The Johns Hopkins Hospital in Baltimore. It was exactly eleven years since I heard the chilling words, "We found spots." John, who is more a brother to me than a cousin, is lying in bed, unable to speak, fighting a rare form of leukemia.

Eyes almost closed, he motions me over and tries to speak. I look at his wife Michelle and say softly, "I can't understand what he's saying." Michelle, by now already fluent in his silent communication, responds with a lovely smile: "He says he's Spartan strong." John hears her and gives me the thumbs-up sign. We press our foreheads together.

Being with John has jolted me. It feels like his struggle is a direct challenge to me. What have I done with my experience to help others? How had I managed to bury all those emotions and experiences that needed to be shared?

Being with John not only brings back all of my cancer related feelings, but gives me the resolve to speak up about them with others. However, if I'm going to share these difficult, raw emotions, I must re-learn how to embrace them and not rush to cover them up or numb them out.

Eleven years after cancer treatment, I still experience occasional sharp pains about two inches above my right ear. Perhaps they are the aftershocks of all that chemo and radiation. In any case, they are an accepted part of my life, useful reminders of what I experienced and the importance of valuing each day. I have recovered the ability to be present in the moment. I can accept the uncertainty of the future. I am alive right now and that's more than enough reason to be happy.

PART II: THE EXERCISES

The Benefits of Exercise

The exercise program I developed while undergoing chemotherapy was crucial to my recovery. It provided three major benefits—strength, control, and confidence.

First, it gave me the physical and mental strength to endure the arduous treatments without becoming completely worn out. In fact, I believe my workouts allowed me to stay one step ahead of my medical care instead of just limping from one procedure to the next. For example, I sometimes felt strong enough to endure a few tests in a single day, allowing me to avoid multiple hour-long trips into the city.

I vividly remember the day I was fitted for the mask I would wear during radiation treatments. It was a very stressful procedure in which my entire face was covered for forty-five minutes with only two small holes open at my nostrils to allow me to breathe. To get through the ordeal, I calmed myself by thinking about the meditative breathing I had been doing as part of my daily exercise routine.

When it was over, they needed to schedule a spinal tap to see if any cancer cells had entered my spine. "Can I do it today?" I asked. I didn't want to make another trip to the hospital and felt strong enough to go ahead. They agreed. That proved to be even worse than the mask-fitting. The pressure I felt when the needle entered my spine was unlike anything I'd ever experienced. But, again, I believe the exercise routine gave me the resilience to take it in stride.

Second, the workout program gave me a greater sense of control over my life and aided my ability to become an active manager of my treatment program instead of a passive recipient.

It helped reinforce my conviction that all patients should ask questions whenever they are confused or uncertain about the steps recommended by medical professionals. For me, the key "ask questions!" moment came when I was told that a port would be planted in my chest to receive IV chemotherapy. I objected because I worried that my son, Benjamin, would be freaked out by it. "Aren't there other options?" I asked. With some persistence, they agreed to use needles every time they needed to hook up an IV. Although they warned me my veins might collapse, I'm convinced my cancer treatment exercise program was vital to keeping my veins strong and accessible, able to endure more than a hundred injections.

I'm not suggesting that other cancer patients should resist having a port. For them, it may be the best option. My point is simply that patients need to be their own advocate. You may not always get what you want, but you do have the right to know about your options.

The third great benefit of exercise was the greater confidence it gave me about my prospects for recovery, a confidence that in turn spread to my loved ones. They could see my exercise program was giving me a better ability to cope with my situation and that gave them the ability to be more comfortable and normal in my company and communicate honestly (as opposed to walking around on egg shells).

I was especially aware of this benefit when I attended Benjamin's weekend basketball games. Walking into that gym, I felt many eyes looking my way. It's a small town and news of my cancer was well established. But for Benjamin's sake, and my own, I wanted those afternoons to be as normal as possible, with attention on the game, not on my health. I would sit next to Alan, Benjamin's grandfather, and we would root on Benjamin's team. After the game, Benjamin did not ask how I was doing, but only what I thought of the game and how he had played. My own enhanced confidence in public, aided by my exercise program, helped Benjamin live through these months in a much more settled way.

Strength, control, confidence—all were greatly enhanced by my workout routine. This book is an effort to share my experience so it might benefit other people who have been recently diagnosed with cancer. I believe it also can help friends and family members who want to be as supportive as possible. In addition, this program will be useful to medical experts who already are beginning to recognize the benefits of exercise during cancer treatment. The goal is to provide actionable skills that will develop the physical strength and flexibility and psychological control to help people transcend the scary reality of life with cancer. You will come away with a new appreciation for your body and mind working in sync to save one another.

Flipping Your Switch

My exercise routine evolved out of an intuition that challenging my body would improve my chances of returning to full health. I had the benefit of always enjoying exercise, but that did not drive this experience. My primary inspiration was my son Benjamin. I vividly remember telling myself that if I could just survive until he graduated from high school he would be fine. I saw exercise as the primary thing I could do to improve my odds.

I believe moderate exercise can help every cancer patient. Of course, cancer treatments vary widely, as do the side-effects. For example, not all cancer patients undergo chemotherapy and those who do receive many different kinds of drugs via delivery systems ranging from intravenous drips to pills and injections.

Whatever the treatment protocol, we all have our low moments when we feel especially tired and lacking in motivation. For me, that happened after every cycle of chemo. I would return home from the hospital feeling exhausted. My routine was to head straight to the couch and collapse. Typically, I would stay there for a good twenty-four hours rising only for the bare essentials. At that point, I always made a conscious decision to get up and renew my exercise routine. Otherwise, I might be tempted to just remain sunk into my couch cushions.

The first move was simply to swing my legs over the couch and stand up. To this day, that two-legged swing is by far the hardest thing I have ever asked my body to do. I felt like I was lifting myself out of a safe nest to answer the boxer's bell, seeing my adversary across the ring prepared and ready to defeat me.

Everyone reacts differently to treatment, both mentally and physically. Regardless, there will be defining moments when you will need your mind to be strong enough to demand that your body begin to exercise. Once that key decision is made, and made repeatedly throughout your treatment, your mind and body will become mutually reinforcing and connected on the same path toward recovery.

For most of our lives our willpower has led the way in teaching us many new things, even when other parts of us cried out, "No, don't do it." Learning to ride a bicycle as a child is one example. To gain that skill, you have to overcome the fear of falling, even when the learning process invariably produces falls. Somehow, we develop the confidence that the falls will become less and less common. What provides that confidence? Partly, it's sheer determination. But mostly it's the exhilaration that comes when your parent releases the back of the seat and yells, "Pedal!" Suddenly your body is shot through with endorphins and adrenalin that help suppress your fears and trigger your body to do its job—to keep pedaling while trying to balance the bike as you move forward. The gradually gained ability to ride longer and longer distances without stopping or falling keeps building your confidence and your exhilaration at the new-found freedom of mobility. When it all clicks, it's almost like magic, mind and body working as one so you don't even have to think about it anymore.

Now is the time for your mind to help your body fight. You need to push yourself to get on that "bike" and pedal like your life depends on it—because it does.

Psychological Benefits of Exercise

Dr. Katherine Appy is a clinical psychologist whose practice includes individuals (and their loved ones) at every stage of cancer treatment. She draws on a wide range of psychotherapeutic approaches that encourage patients to become more conscious of mind-body connections and their relationship to health. Here is what she has to say about the benefits of exercising while in treatment:

"When you are diagnosed with cancer you are likely to feel anxious, fearful, and depressed. You may also feel a host of other emotions, some of them unexpected and even positive. A regular routine of exercise, as practiced and advocated by Peter Green, can help you reduce negative feelings and gain a greater sense of control over your life. Peter discovered that exercise not only greatly contributed to his recovery, but helped his loved ones interact with him in more open and hopeful ways.

Feeling better about yourself during cancer treatment also helps you relate to those who care about you. Family and friends are often unsure what to say or how to act in your presence. You may feel compelled to put on a happy face to reduce their fear and anxiety. When others observe your real feelings and a growing sense that you're taking control, they are also less likely to pretend emotions they don't feel. It paves the way for more authentic support.

Many studies have found a strong link between exercise and mood. Among other benefits, exercise helps the body release endorphins—our own natural brain chemicals that enhance both physical and psychological well-being. Staying as fit as possible also helps maintain self-esteem while at the same time reducing stress.

Exercise raises your heart rate and makes you sweat—the same things that happen when people feel great anxiety! One fascinating study demonstrates that people who exercise regularly are more likely to associate rapid pulse and sweat with safety and health rather than fear and anxiety, thus enhancing their ability to deal with difficult feelings.

The greater confidence that comes with exercise may also move you to take other helpful steps. You might be more likely to join a cancer support group, begin psychotherapy, seek out trusted friends, or open yourself to new or long abandoned practices such as meditation and mindfulness. All these things can increase your feelings of well-being and connection.

Exercise can be central to your efforts to take control of the fear, anxiety and depression that often accompany a cancer diagnosis."

The Science of Cancer Treatment Workouts

Exercise and its relationship to cancer is a burgeoning field of study. Although most research so far has focused on the effects of exercise on cancer prevention, new information has begun to emerge on exercise during cancer treatment that show genuine benefits. They include:

1. Improved body and weight management. Builds muscle, trims fat.

2. Maintenance or improvement of cardiovascular fitness. Builds endurance.

3. Mobility / flexibility. Makes your body more pliable and resilient.

4. Develops mindfulness, a greater ability to focus on the moment.

5. Helps reduce anxiety, depression and other emotional pitfalls.

Maintaining movement and physical activity throughout cancer treatment has also been found to produce many specific physiological effects:

1. Raises the level of cancer-fighting antioxidants.

2. Improves the body's ability to fight inflammation.

3. Stimulates healthy cell metabolism.

4. Aids in recovery from the debilitating side-effects of chemotherapy and radiation. One study found that patients who "exercised regularly had 40% to 50% less fatigue, the primary complaint during treatment."

5. Some animal and human studies show it can even reduce the size and number of malignant tumors.

There is also growing evidence that people who exercise during treatment are able to complete more chemotherapy sessions than those who do not exercise.

FAQ

Shouldn't I just rest to give my body the best chance to heal?

You do need to rest, especially just after each treatment cycle. But exercise improves the quality of your rest and your sleep. When you relax or sleep after exercise, your body rebuilds itself from the stimulation of deep breathing, cardiovascular exertion, and resistance training. Your body will get stronger, not weaker, and better able to recover. Exercise will help give you the physical and mental strength and endurance to counteract the weakening ordeal of chemotherapy or radiation.

Won't exercise exhaust me and make me more vulnerable to other illnesses?

Quite the opposite. It is a medical fact that the right kind of exercises build your immune system, making you stronger and less susceptible to other illnesses. Of course, since cancer treatments often lower white cell counts, patients must be careful about exposing themselves to people and places that carry disease. However, doing moderate exercise in the safety of your own home does not put you at risk. In fact, it will stimulate blood flow, increase range of motion, release endorphins, all of which will enhance your physical and emotional well-being.

How can I do these exercises if I haven't worked out much in the past?

This exercise program is designed for people at all levels of physical fitness. It also takes into account the physical and emotional stress caused by cancer treatment. Many of the motions required by these exercises are as common as everyday life—raising your arms over your head, standing up, and so on. Also, you can modify the number of repetitions you do, or the weight of the ball you use, to match the level of challenge best suited for you. The main point is to do whatever you can with focus, good form, and conscious breathing. It should be as much a meditation as a workout.

Will I need a trainer to do these workouts?

No. All the exercises are simple and straightforward. Detailed instructions are provided for each one and after doing them a few times you will easily remember how to do them.

Should I consult with my oncologist before beginning this exercise program?

Yes. Your doctor may have some useful advice on the level of exercise best-suited to you. However, always remember that it's your life and you have the final say on what you do with your body. You're the one who has cancer and sometimes your instincts about what you need to do can and should overrule the professionals.

Basic Equipment

1 Yoga/exercise mat

2 A 2-lb. Pilate's ball and a 4-lb. weight ball. Begin with the lighter ball as you learn the exercises and develop proper form. While using the heavier ball, if your form becomes sloppy or your breathing strained, switch to the lighter ball.

3 Elastic exercise bands. The standard progression from lightest to heaviest resistance is: yellow, green, red, blue, black.

I. Foundational Exercises

Exercise Type: Mind-Body

Purpose: Preparation, Focus, Breath control, Trunk stability, Body awareness, Core strength, Spinal mobility

Intensity: Low

Frequency: Every day

As you learn the exercises be sure to focus on your breathing. Establishing proper breath control is essential to making your workouts as productive as possible. You should listen to your breathing to be sure it is working in harmony with your body. Always inhale during the least stressful part of each exercise and exhale during the most arduous. For example, when you do the chest press with a weight ball, you should inhale when you bring the ball down to your chest. This is the recovery part of the exercise and the least stressful. Take as much air as you need, but try to inhale through your nose. As you push the ball up begin to exhale gradually through your mouth. This is the most difficult part of the exercise.

It sounds like a small thing, but breathing correctly is the most important part of every exercise. It allows your body to work with maximum efficiency and strength and to recover fully for the next major exertion.

The Angel Stretch

- Lie on your back with knees bent about 45 degrees and feet flat.
- Put your hands at your side, palms up.

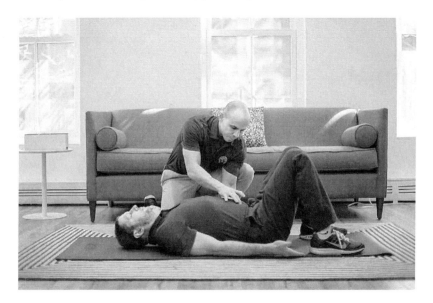

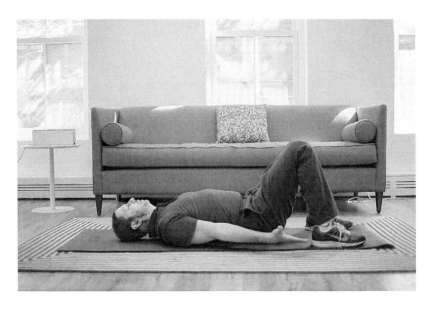

- Slowly move both arms out to the side, just above the floor and over your head. (Just like a "snow angel").

- Keep the palms up and hands as close to the floor as possible without touching the floor.

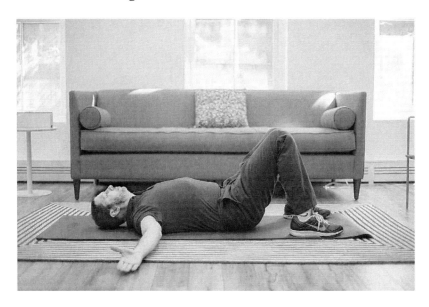

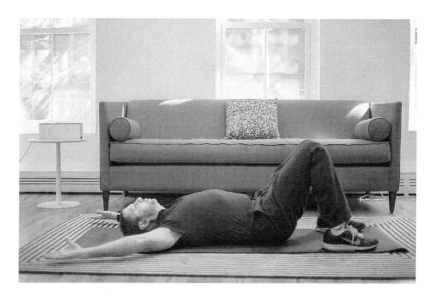

- Bring your thumbs and forefingers together in the shape of a diamond.

- Gently exhale and tighten your abdominal muscles. Feel the small of your back pressed to the floor.

- Now, raise your straight arms over your head until you can look up and see through the diamond of your fingers before beginning the process again.

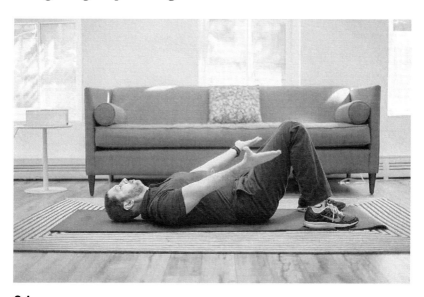

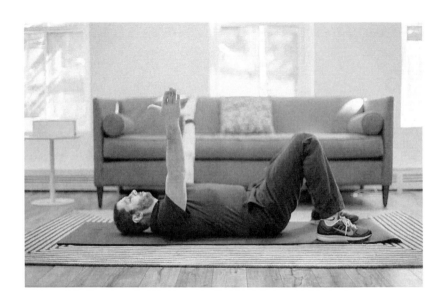

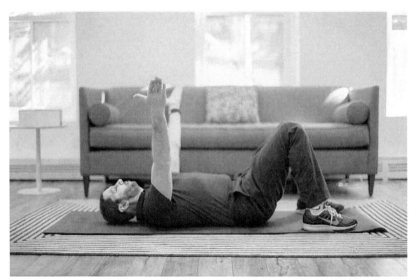

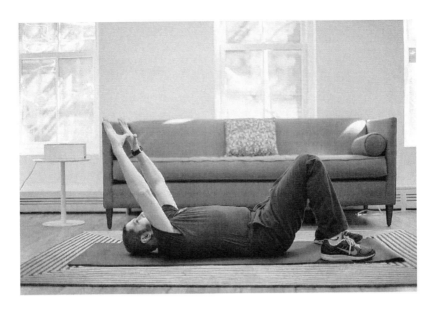

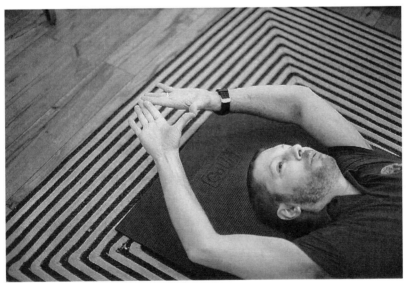

- Slowly bring your hands down over your mouth and exhale through the space. Now, raise your hands back up until your arms are fully extended.

- Once your arms are fully extended, with the space directly over your eyes, slowly bring your hands back down to your sides, palms up, just off the surface of the mat.

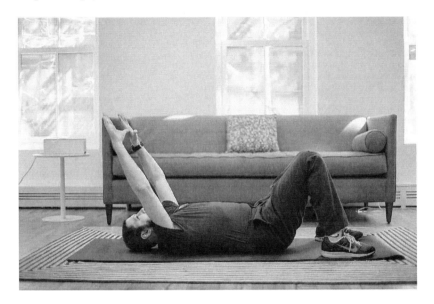

- Repeat the entire stretch with eyes closed. This removes one sense, while enhancing the others. With eyes closed you will become more acutely aware of your breathing, your stretching muscles and the movement of your arms. The angel stretch is a meditative exercise. With your eyes closed you may see vivid colors.

Core Exercises

Strengthening your core, building your strength. Foundational exercises of the trunk, spine and core muscles are vital to the cancer treatment workout program. Trunk and core exercises provide multiple benefits including:

- Body awareness
- Muscle control
- Muscle strength and endurance
- Spinal mobility

Core 1: Trunk Stability

INSTRUCTIONS

- Lie on your back with knees bent about 45 degrees and feet flat.
- Put your hands at your side, palms up.
- Press the small of your back against the floor.
- Slowly arch your back two inches off the floor. Inhale as you raise the small of your back; exhale as you lower your back.
- Repeat 3-10 times.

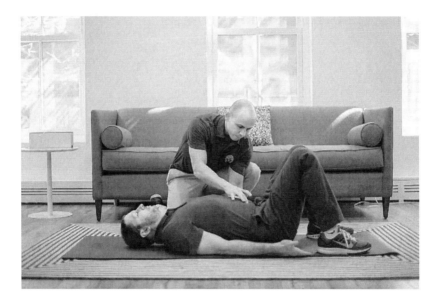

Core 2: Hip Lifts

- Lie on your back with knees bent about 45 degrees and feet flat.

- Use your leg and abdominal muscles to raise your hips 6-8 inches off the floor.

- Keep your feet and shoulders firmly planted on the floor. Hold your hips up for 3 breaths.

- Slowly lower your hips to the ground.

- Repeat 3-10 times.

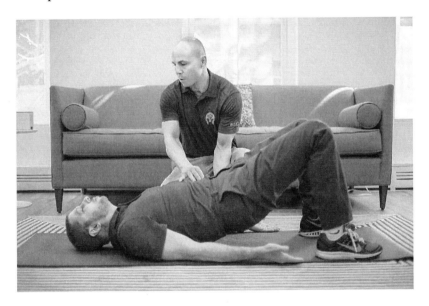

Core 3: Hip Drops

- Get on your hands and knees with your arms and thighs straight and your back flat. Keep head in neutral position.

- Drop your hips back over your heels while keeping back flat and arms stretched out forward.

- Take two, easy breaths. Engage abdominal muscles and move hips forward to the original position. Keep head and spine in the neutral position.

- Repeat 10 times.

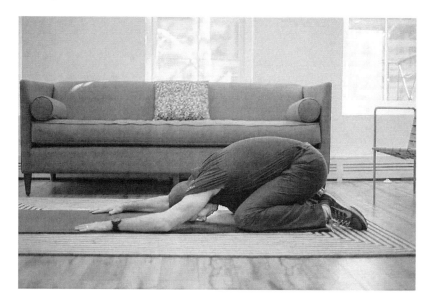

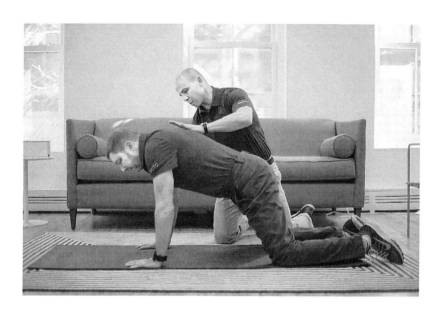

II: Resistance Training

Exercise type: Strength building

Purpose: Overall physical and mental strength and endurance

Intensity: Low/Moderate

Frequency: Two or Three times a week

WEIGHT BALL/ELASTIC BAND EXERCISES

Once the cycle of foundational exercises has been completed you are ready to move into weight ball (either a 2-lb. Pilate's ball or a 4-lb. weight ball) and elastic band exercises. Start light, even without a ball, to perfect the motions. Small weight ball exercises are a safe alternative to dumbbells. A ball also allows for more freedom of movement and necessitates hand strength and coordination.

Complete the following exercises as a circuit after the angel stretch and core exercises. Performing the exercises as a circuit will reduce local fatigue and generate total body blood flow and nerve activation.

Once you introduce the ball, 3-10 repetitions of each movement are recommended based on your current level of function. Ultimately, aim for 10 reps per exercise and two sets of the circuit. Do what you can to start. Keep in mind it is not necessary to perform all of the exercises. Only perform the movements you can do comfortably and with good form.

1. Chest Press

- Lie on your mat with knees up and feet firmly on the ground.
- Mildly engage your trunk by keeping the small of you back against the floor.
- Hold the weight ball with both hands just above your chest.
- Slowly exhale as you lift the ball straight up.
- With your arms fully extended, inhale and lower the ball to your chest.
- Repeat 3-10 repetitions

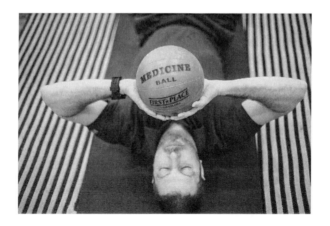

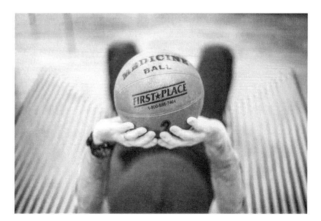

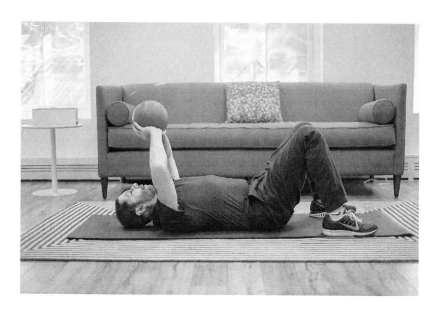

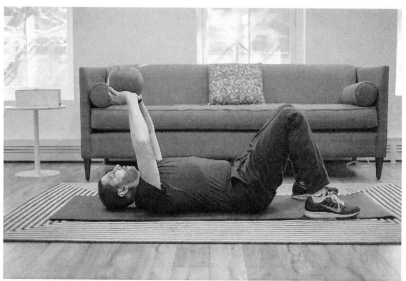

2. One Arm Press

- Lie on your mat with knees up and feet firmly on the ground.
- Mildly engage your trunk by keeping the small of you back against the floor.
- Hold the weight ball in one hand above your chest. Begin with very light ball.
- The hand that does not have the ball should be lightly placed across your chest or abdomen.
- Slowly exhale as you lift the ball straight up.
- With your arms fully extended, inhale and lower the ball to your chest.
- 3-10 repetitions for each hand.

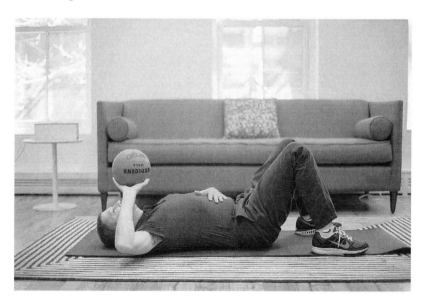

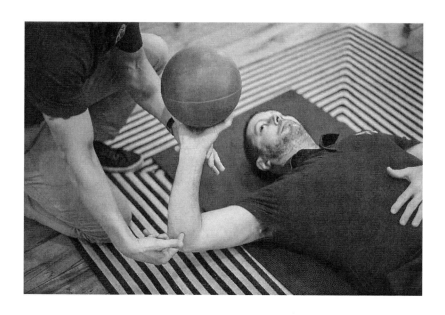

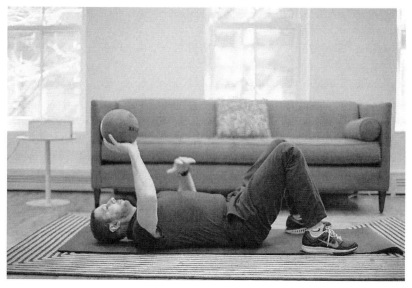

3. Weight Ball Hand Passes

- Begin in the same position: on back with knees up and feet flat.
- Raise the ball up with one hand. Then lift the other arm.
- Once both arms are fully extended, rotate the ball and hand it off to your empty hand and slowly lower the ball.
- 3-10 repetitions each side.

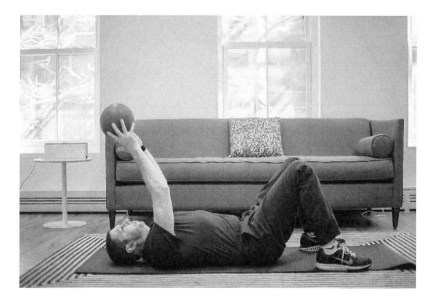

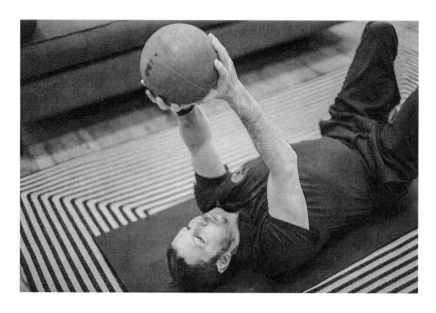

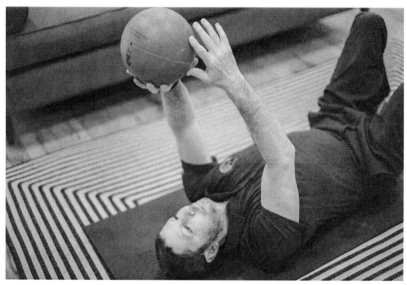

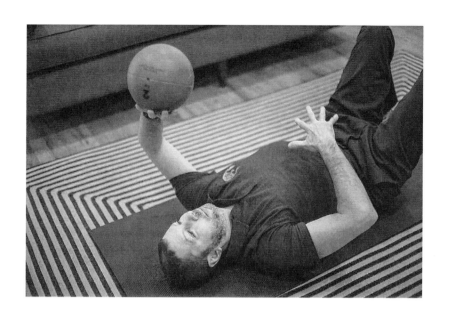

4. Band Pulls

- Either stand up with your feet at shoulder width, or sit upright in chair.

- Grip the middle of the band with both hands, about 12 inches apart, palms down.

- Raise the band to shoulder height. With arms straight out, stretch the band outward to each side. Keep your shoulders down and gently squeeze the shoulder blades together.

- Slowly allow the band to rebound and drop your arms to your waist.

- 3-10 repetitions.

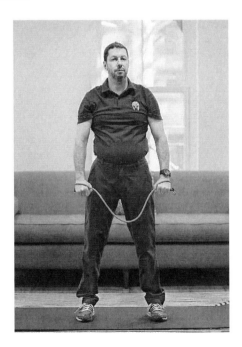

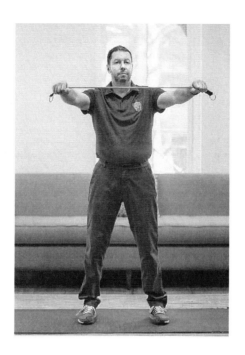

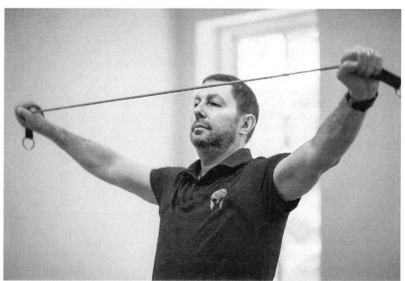

5. Sit-to-Stand

INSTRUCTIONS

- Start in a seated position on a stable chair, or standing with your feet flat on the floor. Optional: Hold a weight ball in your lap.

- Maintain a good posture and rise to a standing position by using your leg muscles.

- Keep your abdomen engaged throughout the movement.

- If you have trouble with balance or leg strength, bring you nose over your toes when you begin the movement. Keep your back straight.

- If your balance is very poor, have a spotter hold your hands or elbows. You may also hold onto a nearby object such as a table or shelf.

- Return to the seated position by slowly lowering your body by squatting (reach your hips and buttocks backward to sit). Maintain your posture and abdominal tension.

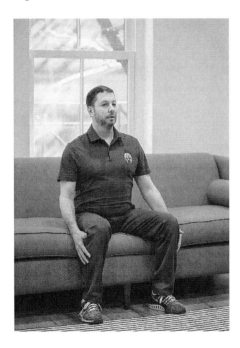

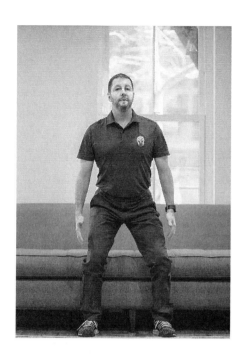

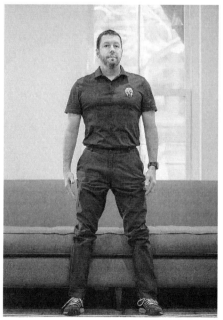

6. Ball Curls

- Stand with your feet at shoulder width and elbows tucked to your side with knees slightly bent (you may also perform this exercise in a seated position)
- With the ball in both hands, palms up, slowly bring the ball from the elbow position upward in a controlled motion.
- Keep your abdominal muscles engaged and maintain good posture.
- Exhale as you flex your arms upward.
- Slowly return to the starting position.
- 3-10 repetitions.

Option: Instead of a weight ball, you can do curls with a resistance band (holding the band under one foot, or two). Or, you could rotate between the ball and the band on alternate workout days.

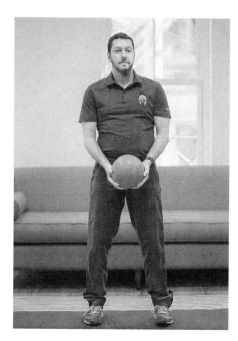

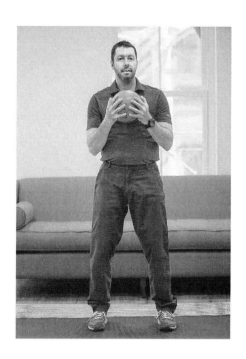

7. Forearm Rolls

INSTRUCTIONS

- Begin in the same position you use for ball curls.

- Using a 2-lb. Pilates ball, lift and roll your forearm, slowly transferring the ball from one hand to the other, keeping elbows in against your body.

- 3-10 repetitions.

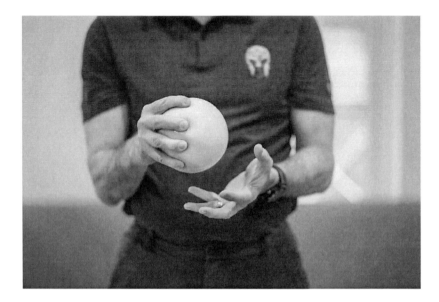

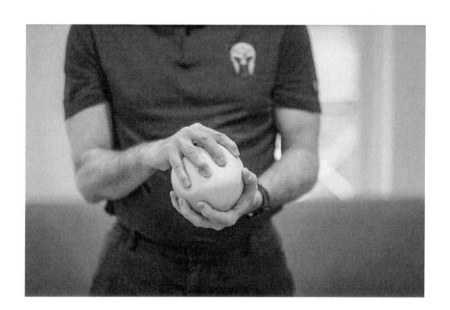

8. Tennis Ball Squeeze
(FREE TIME SUPPLEMENT TO FOREARM ROLLS)

INSTRUCTIONS

- Just squeeze a tennis ball while you're watching television or talking with friends. If a tennis ball is too firm, try a soft "stress ball," or putty.

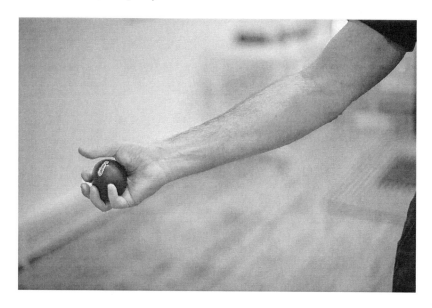

Sometimes the simplest exercises are the best! When I was training for the Peace Corps in South Carolina, I broke a thumb playing football with friends. I was sent to a Marine Corps doctor at nearby Parris Island where the Marines train. A few weeks later, when the doctor finally buzzed off my cast, there was no coddling. He simply told me to wash off my limp arm in a sink and then he tossed me a tennis ball. "Squeeze this for a couple of weeks and you'll be fine." He was right. It's one of the best ways to build hand and forearm strength. You can also bounce it off the floor and catch it, a fun exercise that helps your reflexes.

9. The Wall Pillar

The Wall Pillar exercise is a total body exercise that establishes stability, balance, and control.

INSTRUCTIONS

- Stand facing a wall with your arms fully extended in front of you with palms against the wall (as if you were going to do a push-up).
- Your feet should be about two feet away from the wall, and shoulder width apart.
- With head up, and eyes focused straight ahead at the wall, gently engage your abdomen.
- Slowly lift one knee until your leg forms a 90-degree angle. Hold the position for one second and then slowly lower your leg.
- Now do the same with your other knee.
- It should feel like slow-motion marching.
- 3-10 repetitions with each leg.

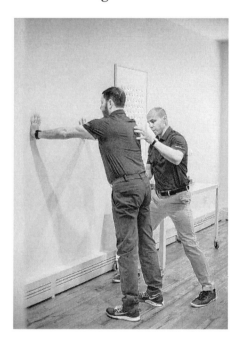

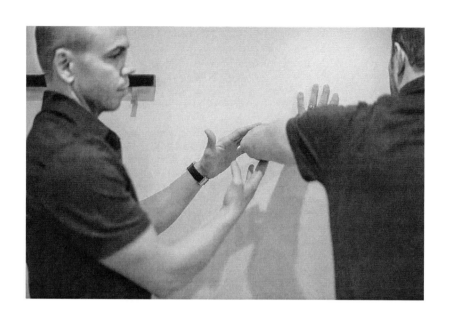

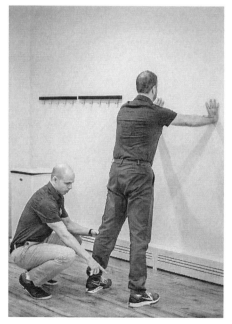

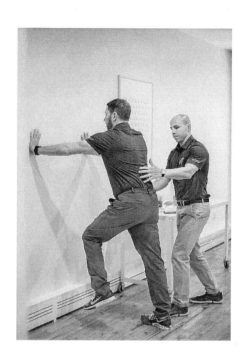

III. Aerobic Exercise

Exercise type: Cardiovascular

Purpose: To build physical and mental endurance

Intensity: Low to Moderate (No more than 65% of maximum heart rate.

To calculate your max heart rate, subtract your age from 220.

Then determine the percentage you want to reach. Example: 220 minus age 50 equals 170. Sixty-five percent of 170 is 110 (max heart rate for 50-year-old cancer patient)

Frequency: Low intensity aerobic exercise (e.g., walking) can be performed every day

Aerobic exercise involves any rhythmic or repetitive movement performed at low to moderate intensity. If performed frequently health benefits can be realized in as little as 5-10 minutes. Examples of aerobic activity include walking, running, cycling, swimming, rowing, and various cardio machines (i.e., the elliptical). Aerobic exercise also can be performed in short, highly intense, intervals followed by short recovery times. However, I believe interval training puts too much stress on the cardiovascular and pulmonary systems to be advisable during cancer treatments. My research has convinced me that low intensity exercise offers the best chance for achieving fitness during this crucial time.

Epilogue

It's been 12 years since I heard the words, "We found something." For more than a decade I chose not to confront my feelings about my struggles with brain cancer. However, while writing this book, I realized the fears I felt, the transitions that were happening in my life and ultimately finding the courage to fight, I now choose to deal with every day. This is my life. I'm no longer a silent bystander, but someone who has taken control of their own destiny.

The result of which is the launch of my company, Workout Through Cancer LLC www.workoutthroughcancer.com. My goal is to take all the feelings I experienced and build a community that not only permits those emotions to come to the surface, but to find ways to overcome them.

I heard a quote recently which began, "Some beginnings are endings and some endings are beginnings," which got me thinking. For me, there are no endings or beginnings, only movement of one's energy that evolves and creates continual movement.

There is nothing pretty about cancer. It is a brutal disease that rips at the fabric of so many lives. Families are destroyed, dreams are never realized, and careers come to an abrupt stop. Yet, for me, as strange as it sounds, I never felt as alive as when I was going through my struggle and this is what I am beginning to feel again—a purpose.

My story does not end here. Hopefully, it will continue to expand and I will be able to help those with cancer, as well as their families and loved ones, find the inner strength, energy and courage to forge on and fight the good fight.

I don't know where all of this will eventually lead, or if my company will succeed. I do know I can't imagine doing anything else.

ACKNOWLEDGMENTS

Anyone who has survived cancer knows how crucial it is to have supportive friends, colleagues, and medical professionals to count on. I can't mention everyone who gave me support throughout my treatment and recovery and who encouraged my effort to write this book, but I do want to single out Seth Sholes, Jill Benz, Abigail List, Elise Fuchs, Ed Darmanin, Jim Noble, Shieva Ghofrany, Maura Igoe, Phil Alcabes, the Seligson family—Nancy, Alan, Edith and Kate—all my colleagues at the Weather Channel, and the great doctors and staff at Memorial Sloan Kettering Cancer Center.

Special thanks to Josh Lander who, from the start, believed in the exercises I created and how they could help those going through cancer treatment.

Of all my friends I especially want to thank Duke Saltus, a fellow cancer survivor and a trusted friend for more than fifty years. Over almost daily coffee's we have shared all our hopes, frustrations, and the many memories of growing up together.

I am also deeply indebted to the members of my cancer support group at the Smilow Cancer Hospital at the Yale Cancer Center, especially Dr. Marni Amsellem. Their stories and struggles inspire me every time we meet.

This book stresses the great importance of family support for anyone struggling with cancer. I've been blessed with an unusually large and caring family. I want first to thank my four siblings, Andrew, Alex, Doug, and Kathy. Each has played a crucial role in supporting my recovery. Alex came from the West Coast many times to be with Ben and me between treatments and Kathy stayed with me every night in the hospital during many cycles of chemotherapy. I also want to thank my cousin Bill Green and Michelle Green who gave me so much support even as they were going through such a difficult time in their own lives. My step-brother, William Craig, an accomplished writer, encouraged my writing and showed me some tricks of the trade.

At any early stage of work on this book I was helped by developmental editor Richard Marek. Without his encouragement, I would never have had the confidence to continue. I later turned for help to my brother-in-law, Chris Appy, a gifted writer and historian. His painstaking editorial work helped convert my story into a book people may want to read.

I am forever grateful to my parents, Paul Green and Sonya Warshawsky, and my step-mother of forty years, Eleanor Green. Their unconditional love and support has been a constant source of strength and inspiration. Their struggles with Parkinson's and cancer exemplify grace under pressure.

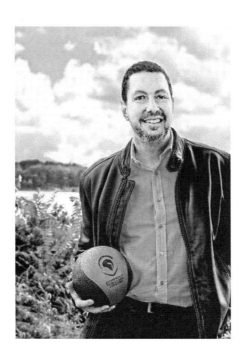

PETER GREEN, founder of "Workout Through Cancer," is a native of Westport, Connecticut. After attending Seattle University, he spent two years with the Peace Corps in West Africa. Later, he launched a successful career in print and digital media with McGraw Hill, *Institutional Investor* magazine, and Weather.com. He's back living in his hometown with his wife, Mary, and two dogs, Max and Louie, and is the proud father of a grown son, Benjamin.